Running on Empty

——————————◆——————————

"The Centers for Disease Control defined Chronic Fatigue Immune Dysfunction Syndrome (CFIDS) in March of 1988. Now, over three years later, very few physicians even believe it exists, and countless people suffer from the disease without knowing what they have or how to deal with it. This comprehensive examination of CFIDS is up-to-date and gives excellent mechanisms for recognizing and coping with this debilitating syndrome. Dr. Berne's book is a current and well researched thesis on what *is* known about CFIDS, how it is diagnosed, and how one can learn to live with the deficits it causes."

David L. Payne, D.O.
CFIDS practitioner and researcher

"I highly recommend RUNNING ON EMPTY. As a physician who has been ill with CFIDS for four years, I find it highly accurate in terms of characteristics of the illness itself and regarding current research in progress. This book is written from the standpoint of both psychologist and patient and is written in a form that makes it readily understandable to the patient. I highly recommend this book to health care providers and patients."

Sara S. Reynolds, M.D., AAFP
Executive Board Member, CFS Association of Arizona

To Mabel
who had stars in her eyes

RUNNING ON EMPTY

Chronic Fatigue Immune Dysfunction Syndrome (CFIDS)

———————◆———————

Katrina H. Berne, Ph.D.

Hunter House

Hunter House Inc., Publishers
2200 Central Avenue, Suite 202
Alameda, CA 94501
Acknowledgement is made for permission to reprint "A Symptom Checklist for CFS" from Chronic Fatigue Syndrome Institute, 500 South Anaheim Hills Road, #128, Anaheim Hills, CA 92807
© Jay A. Goldstein, M.D.

Library of Congress Cataloging-in-Publication Data:
Berne, Katrina.
Running on empty : chronic fatigue immune dysfunction syndrome (CFIDS) / Katrina Berne. — 1st ed.
p. cm.
Includes bibliographical references (p.) and index.
ISBN 0-89793-100-9 : $13.95 — ISBN 0-89793-101-7 : $21.95
1. Chronic fatigue syndrome—Popular works. I. Title.
RB150.F37B47   1991
616'.047—dc20   91-47586
                                                                    CIP

Book design by Qalagraphia
Cover design by Tamra Goris Design, Claremont, CA
Copyediting by Anne Ingram
Editorial Coordination: Corrine M. Sahli and Lisa E. Lee
Production Manager: Paul J. Frindt
Publisher: Kiran S. Rana
Set in 11/13 point Goudy Old Style by 847 Communications, Alameda CA
Printed by Griffin Printing, Sacramento, CA
Manufactured in the United States of America

9   8   7   6   5   4   3   2   1   First edition

Table of Contents

◆

IMPORTANT NOTICE

Acknowledgments

Given my unpredictable and unrelenting health fluctuations, it's amazing I've completed this book, and I couldn't have done it without the support and encouragement of some very helpful and generous people.

My parents, Arthur and Claire Berne, who have seen me through my skinned-knees years and my I'll never-get-through-college woes, have come through again on several fronts, supporting me in so many ways during my illness, doctoral studies, and the writing of this book.

My husband Eldon, who married an unknown quantity (he married me post-onset but pre-diagnosis), has tolerated my mood swings, strange hours, and bizarre treatments (with their accompanying side effects and my complaints); listened to endless litanies on my various theories and ordeals; and weathered alternate declarations that I'll survive and triumph—and that I'll never make it. He has offered feedback, comfort, and consolation, and more love and encouragement than I thought humanly possible.

My kids Karen and Jeffrey, who have continued to have needs of their own (as kids tend to do), have nonetheless tolerated a mother who spent most of her time at work, sick in bed, or writing and swearing at the computer.

Caroline Shrodes offered warmth, encouragement, and wisdom, not to mention help with punctuation. She pushed me to publish—to share my knowledge of CFIDS with others.

Lisa Lee and Corrine Sahli—editorial consultants—and the other wonderful folks at Hunter House have offered encouragement, advice, and most importantly the opportunity to reach others with my work.

I am grateful to the dedicated physicians and other health professionals involved in CFIDS treatment and research who have risked the censure of a skeptical medical establishment to serve the needs of PWCs (persons with CFIDS). I feel very close to other PWCs and wish to offer special thanks to those who have filled out questionnaires, endured interviews that lasted hours, and urged me forward in my work.

I am endlessly grateful to these special people and to the others who have seen me through this far and who will probably stick around for more.

Katrina Berne
Mesa, Arizona 1992

Foreword

Through her own professional and personal experience with Chronic Fatigue Syndrome (CFS or CFIDS), Dr. Berne has developed an intimate and thorough knowledge of the disease. The horror, frustration, and anger produced by the disabling condition are graphically portrayed, yet balanced by the reality of palliative treatment and hope for future research.

Most Americans have heard of CFS, Chronic Epstein-Barr (CEBV), or "yuppie flu," or know someone suffering from the disease. However, the fledgling scientific literature of CFS has reached few patients and even fewer physicians. While patients are acutely aware of the potentially disabling power of the disease, most researchers and physicians continue to view CFS as a trivial anthill on the mountain of medicine.

While scientific research will ultimately yield answers to the many unknowns of CFS, this work is truly a landmark compendium of present knowledge in the field. For the physician, the book presents an historical summary, reviews theories of pathogenesis, and outlines current therapeutic strategies. Additionally, and perhaps more importantly, the author reifies the debilitating, disabling effects of the disease and contradicts the common perception that it is trivial or even nonexistent. Postulated etiologies of the disease challenge medical researchers to intensify their efforts.

Patients are presented with a complete, readable, and comprehensible self-study course in CFIDS. Chapters dedicated to self-help and adjustment to chronic disease are particularly critical for patients suffering from an incurable, long-lasting disease. Common pitfalls of self-diagnosis and self-treatment are clearly illustrated. Families and friends can find insight into the symptoms and reactions to symptoms which alter the physical functioning and personalities of their loved one. The author also suggests realistic and functional solutions to improve interpersonal relationships and to preserve the family structure. An extensive bibliography directs those interested in historic and current publications to scientific and lay literature on CFIDS. Physicians, patients, and their families are provided with a current list of support groups, research organizations, and governmental agencies serving the cause of CFIDS.

Finally, society at large is confronted with the desperate need for recognition of this worldwide health problem. Lack of research funding, lack of national interest on the part of federal and private research agencies, and physician misinformation and apathy combine to retard discovery into the pathogenesis and treatment of the disorder. Hopefully, this book will serve to unite and stimulate a broad base of support and research into CFIDS.

CFIDS is fraught with systematic difficulties including diagnostic and therapeutic confusion due in large part to unknown or unproven etiology and pathogenesis. This creates frustration for the physician as well as the patient and often leads to a dysfunctional and unsatisfactory patient/physician relationship. Dr. Berne strives to look beyond knowledge gaps and expose the poorly defined disease process in terms of its functional impact on the physical and mental health of the patient. Numerous real-life examples compel the physician to accept the seriousness of CFIDS; patients are reassured that they are not alone in the morass of signs and symptoms. The author has intertwined experiential data with hard science to produce the most complete overview of CFIDS to date. It will undoubtedly serve as a catalyst for future research and as a ready reference for patients and families of those suffering from CFIDS.

Daniel L. Peterson, M.D.
Incline Village, Nevada, 1992

Preface

◆

A series of astonishing breakthroughs in medical research is gradually bringing the stark realities of CFIDS to the attention of the media, the general public, and the medical establishment. CFIDS is a devastating and elusive illness that afflicts millions and poses a major public health threat. It is a serious disease of immune dysfunction and neurological impairment that is finally being taken seriously.

The tremendous progress being made by a handful of dedicated CFIDS researchers inspires PWCs (persons with CFIDS) as nothing else can. It validates our disease as a distinct clinical entity and gives us hope that the cause(s) and cure(s) will soon be found. These advances also fill us with deep gratitude and pride. We will be forever grateful to the pioneering CFIDS physicians and researchers who have persevered despite the skepticism and derision of their "peers." And we are very proud that PWCs, their families, and friends are largely responsible for this success. We funded much of the research that is legitimizing CFIDS.

These accomplishments at the cutting edge are encouraging and impressive. But the translation of laboratory and clinical findings into diagnostic tools and effective treatments is painfully slow. CFIDS remains. Much of the medical profession continues to ignore, trivialize, or even "psychologize" CFIDS. And, running on empty, PWCs still have a long way to go.

This book is a comprehensive close-up study of CFIDS written by a true CFIDS insider. Without flinching, Katrina Berne, Ph.D, describes the emotional, physical, and cognitive onslaught of this disease, sharing the knowledge of a seasoned

PWC and a trained psychologist who counsels and lectures on that which she knows much about. She explains both the science and the impact of CFIDS, making a mysterious, invisible disease visible and understandable.

Dr. Berne employs an array of devices to depict life with CFIDS: descriptive metaphors, excerpts from her own personal journal, and compassionate vignettes that tell the tales of other PWCs and their feelings. Her insights into the experience and trauma of CFIDS will touch many chords in people with the disease and those who care for them. And her exploration of what PWCs have lost is riveting and frightening.

There is almost nothing you cherish that CFIDS cannot take away. Your health, your mind, your job, your family, your home, your friends, your identity.... Inevitably, CFIDS disrupts or shreds the script for your life and those sharing it.

Fortunately, Dr. Berne pursues the difficult issue of "How do I live with CFIDS?" with the same vigor, wisdom, sympathy, and humor that she uses to explain the nature of the disease. She catalogues the many methods PWCs have devised to grapple with, endure, and grow from the experience of having CFIDS. Her advice on "what to do" includes an analysis of the medical profession and various approaches to healing, identification of treatment programs and lifestyle adjustments, extensive discussion of coping techniques and changes in life philosophy, open letters between PWCs and significant others, guidance on how to form and facilitate a support group, and lists of other resources.

The tools are here for PWCs, their families, their friends, and even their physicians to develop new scripts.

After reading *Running On Empty* you walk away feeling full. It is authoritative but friendly, personal, and easily accessible. It is a resource for everybody and anybody who has an interest in CFIDS. It is the single most useful book on CFIDS to date.

Marc M. Iverson
President, The CFIDS Association, Inc.
Publisher of *The CFIDS Chronicle*

PART I

Chronic Fatigue Immune Dysfunction Syndrome (CFIDS): What It Is

Chapter 1

◆

An Overview of CFIDS

JANE AWOKE ONE MORNING feeling flu-ish and decided to stay in bed. An active, energetic, "Type A" woman, Jane knew she might feel ill for a few days before returning to her normal responsibilities and activity level, as had always been the case with minor illnesses. She'd either keep going despite the illness, or at most take a few days off before resuming her busy schedule. This time didn't feel any different; she felt a bit off-balance and spacey, as if her head were filled with cotton, and had aching joints, a sore throat, tender lymph nodes, and fatigue. "It's just the flu," she told herself. "A week or so of this and then I'll be fine."

Six months later Jane is still in bed most of the time, knowing now that it wasn't just the flu but a lingering illness that has left her debilitated. Her responsibilities—work and family—aren't being fulfilled as well as she'd like, and her former leisure time activities—jogging, hiking, racquetball, lunches with friends, dinner parties—have dwindled to almost nothing. She is often depressed and wonders if she'll ever feel any better. She's feeling crazy and lazy, since no doctor has been able to diagnose her illness. It has been implied and sometimes suggested outright that what she is experiencing is merely the blues, depression, or an anxiety problem, and Jane is beginning to believe what several doctors have told her: that it is "all in her head." Logically she knows that she would never voluntarily have given up her previous lifestyle—the income, the work she enjoyed, her many leisure activities—just to stay in bed and feel awful. She has to drag herself out of bed even to do the basics, such as minor household chores and personal grooming. She feels guilty for neglecting many of her responsibilities but has found that if she pushes herself to be active and to "take care of business" she usually feels worse. "I don't understand what's happening to me. I'm just not myself anymore. I used to be able to do *everything*—and do it well. I always took care of everything and everyone, and I'm not able to do that anymore." Jane wonders whether her life will ever return to normal and fights the possibility that she may have to adapt to this debilitated state and modify her lifestyle significantly in order to cope. And worse, she doesn't understand why she feels so awful all the time. Jane says, "I can handle anything as long as I understand it and know what I'm up against. This feeling, this illness . . . I just can't make sense out of it. I don't know if it's something I'm doing to myself or something from 'out there' I can't control." She wonders how much "legitimacy" her illness has and how it could have happened to her.

Jennifer has always described herself as a low-energy person, reporting frequent illnesses as a child and even as an adult. "I get everything that's going around," she laments. "Whatever flu bug everyone is getting, I always get it, too. I've had measles, flu, chicken pox, mono . . . . I've just gotten used to it." Her previous allergies are now worse, as is her already-low energy level. Over a period of time, Jennifer has felt more and more fatigued. She is now completely unable to work and is fighting the maze of paperwork that accompanies her attempt to obtain disability benefits. But she has no choice: Jennifer is now incapable of working, even part-time, and her self-esteem has plummeted along with her ability to live a "normal" life. "I don't get it. I've been sick a lot—but never this sick, and never for so long." Jennifer has been to a number of doctors and has finally found one who is familiar with her illness, which is called **Chronic Fatigue Syndrome (CFS), or Chronic Fatigue Immune Dysfunction Syndrome (CFIDS).**

CFIDS may be a new problem or a modern version of an illness that has occurred in outbreaks for well over a century. However, it remains a poorly understood illness. It is a disease of immunological and neurological dysfunction, and its cause may be viral. At one time it was called "Chronic Epstein-Barr Virus Syndrome," but this name is no longer used since the Epstein-Barr virus is no longer believed to be the causative agent. Many physicians and patients feel that the name Chronic Fatigue Syndrome trivializes the illness, making it seem like a "crazy and lazy" phenomenon. Walter Gunn, Ph.D., chief CFIDS researcher for the Centers for Disease Control (CDC) said, "The term Chronic Fatigue Syndrome is demeaning to the people who have it," adding that a new name is needed but that at present we have no basis for an appropriate name (November 1991). The term is also inappropriate in that it names a disease after only one of its prominent symptoms (like calling cancer "weight loss syndrome"). The term Chronic Fatigue Immune Dysfunction Syndrome (CFIDS) has come into common usage since it includes the immune abnormalities that have been found in many PWCs (Persons With Chronic Fatigue Immune Dysfunction Syndrome). Several researchers and advocates have suggested that the "F" word be dropped from the name since fatigue is not necessarily the primary characteristic of the illness. Other names have been suggested, such as Chronic Immune Activation Syndrome (coined by Jay Levy, 1990) but a satisfactory and more credible name will probably not be used until the cause of the illness is found. Suspects for the causative agent(s)—there may be more than one—include retroviruses, herpesviruses, adenoviruses, and other infectious agents. But not everyone exposed to the causative agent(s) will necessarily develop the disease. Current research suggests that the onset of CFIDS is a multicausal event, including not only a triggering agent (viral or otherwise), but other factors including age, sex, exposure to environmental toxins, a stressful lifestyle and/or a period of intense stress or work, prior surgery or illness, and immunological defects.

CFIDS is believed to be both an endemic and an epidemic phenomenon; that is, isolated cases are believed to exist in the general population at all times with epidemic outbreaks (affecting thousands or millions of people) occurring periodically. Although such outbreaks have occurred for more than a hundred years, it is not known if the current epidemic is identical to or similar to past outbreaks. Descriptions of earlier outbreaks match the current illness definition quite well but have been poorly documented. Because each outbreak was given a name, noted briefly in the medical literature, and then dismissed, we lack sufficient information to draw solid conclusions. And to further complicate the matter, in examining the current epidemic we may be looking at a number of similar illnesses that fall under one "umbrella."

There are pockets of CFIDS across the United States and in other countries as well—CFIDS is literally all over the map. CFIDS crosses all barriers—age, nationality, gender, income, lifestyle, and occupation—although certain predisposing factors make some people more susceptible than others.

The onset of CFIDS is abrupt in about 75% of cases: most patients can pinpoint exactly when they became ill. "I was sitting in the airport the day before Thanksgiving when I suddenly started to feel awful," says Tom. "My flight was fine, but I wasn't; I don't even remember the time I spent with my relatives. I slept through the entire visit." In other cases, like Jennifer's, the onset is gradual and symptoms appear over an extended period of time.

Female PWCs outnumber males by a 2:1 or 3:1 ratio. This phenomenon is not uncommon in autoimmune diseases, which CFIDS may indeed be. "What are *you* doing with a *woman's* disease?" asked one insensitive doctor of a male PWC. In fact, CFIDS may be less frequently diagnosed among males because men often do not seek medical attention when they are ill. If the "sex bias" does exist it may be explained by hormonal differences and/or occupational differences, since women tend to choose professions in which they have contact with large numbers of people. The majority of known cases occur among professionals, health care workers, airline personnel, and businesspeople, while blue-collar workers and those in solitary professions seem to be least affected, according to Paul Cheney,

M.D. (May 1991). Others are not exempt, however. "CFS is an Equal Opportunity Attacker," wrote Dennis Jackson, Ph.D. (Spring 1991). A few studies comparing healthy individuals and PWCs indicate that their socioeconomic status and educational levels were about the same.

The average age at onset is 37, and most patients are in their middle or "prime" years in the 25–50 age range, hence the nickname "the gray plague" coined by Andrea Blaugrund (1989). Numerous studies indicate that about 75% of patients are aged 20–49; 50–60% are 30–49. The preponderance of cases in these middle, normally productive years is potentially devastating to our work force. However, the age range may be skewed because the illness is probably underdiagnosed in children and perhaps in the elderly as well. CFIDS is found in every age group.

Symptoms vary widely among patients and tend to fall into three general categories: neurological, general or physical, and emotional. Many of the symptoms have been experienced by healthy individuals from time to time, but in PWCs the symptoms are more continuous, severe, and pronounced. In addition, symptoms vary in severity and change over time. A college professor who was forced by CFIDS to take early retirement calls it "the disease of jumping symptoms." Another PWC notes, "The fatigue, dysequilibrium, and frequent illnesses that plagued me in the first year of my illness aren't such a problem anymore. But I now have more difficulty with allergies, digestive problems, and sometimes muscle pain. I'm ill all the time, but the severity and the symptoms keep changing. It's really hard to plan anything or live any kind of predictable life with this crazy stuff going on. I'm getting really angry and fed up, and so is my family. We never know what to expect."

General or **physical symptoms** include: debilitating fatigue; sore throat; swollen or tender lymph nodes; frequent infections; unusual and often severe headaches; allergies (worsening of previous allergies and/or new allergies and sensitivities to foods, odors or chemicals); weight change, usually a gain unaccompanied by a change in eating habits; muscle or joint aches; gastrointestinal problems such as gas, diarrhea, nausea, and abdominal pain; rashes; low grade fevers; night sweats; frequent canker sores; shortness of breath with exertion; heart palpitations; chest pain; cough; urinary tract problems; decreased sex drive.

Neurological symptoms include: sensitivity to bright light; balance problems; "spaceyness" and disorientation; difficulty with concentration and memory; impaired calculation and word-finding abilities; numbness or tingling feelings; sleep disturbance; visual problems; seizure-like episodes, or "blackouts"; unusual and disturbing nightmares; altered spatial perception which is often most evident when driving a vehicle. These neurological symptoms are a hallmark of CFIDS.

Emotional problems associated with CFIDS include: depression, which may be accompanied by suicidal ideation or attempts; anxiety with or without panic attacks; mood swings; a tendency to overreact to minor events. The depression may be both endogenous (chemically caused), and exogenous (caused by external events—in this case, being chronically ill). Although patients often *feel* crazy, many of the emotional changes they experience are directly caused by the illness. Most did not experience such problems prior to the onset of CFIDS.

PWCs generally feel poorly understood by others, experiencing self-doubt as well as relationship conflicts. It is impossible for those without CFIDS to understand the true impact of the illness and the havoc it can wreak on a person's life. Because patients invariably appear healthier than they feel, those with whom they come into contact are not immediately aware of CFIDS-related limitations and often expect the PWC to behave "normally"—that is, to be active and to handle the same responsibilities as in the past. It is difficult for PWCs to communicate the degree of their physical impairment and emotional pain to others, and as a result many relationships are disrupted. In addition, the PWC copes daily with lowered self-esteem, a very restricted activity level, an inability to predict health fluctuations, and a sense of powerlessness and worthlessness due to the inability to function as in the past. Many have based their self-esteem on *what* they were able to do rather than on *who* they were and are, leading to changing roles and identity problems that must be addressed. The emotional fallout of CFIDS can be as devastating as the syndrome itself.

There is no laboratory test to diagnose CFIDS. Diagnosis is based upon symptoms, length of the illness, degree of impairment, and by ruling out other illnesses with similar symptoms. In the past an Epstein-Barr antibody test was used, but this should no longer be regarded as a diagnostic tool since the elevations of Epstein-Barr virus antibodies found in most patients are now viewed as an epiphenomenon rather than a cause of CFIDS. Many PWCs see a large number of doctors before being diagnosed. CFIDS is both underdiagnosed (when patients' symptoms are not understood or taken seriously by their doctors) and overdiagnosed (when fatigue is caused by other factors, including anemia, sleep disorders, psychological/psychiatric disorders, effects of drugs, metabolic disorders, and other chronic illnesses).

The severity of the illness varies considerably among patients as well as in individual patients across time. Some are mildly affected and can carry on a somewhat modified schedule of activities, but others are totally debilitated and disabled. Those in the latter group are generally unable to work and are often confined to bed. Most cases fall between these extremes, with the illness following a waxing and waning cycle.

The Centers for Disease Control, initially resistant to acknowledging the existence of this illness, issued a definition and symptom criteria for the diagnosis of Chronic Fatigue Syndrome (the term they prefer) in March 1988. CFIDS researchers, medical practitioners, and patients agree that their definition is quite narrow in scope and needs to be updated.

The mode of transmission is unknown. Multiple cases of CFIDS in families are not uncommon, and those afflicted are usually genetically related (blood relatives) rather than nonblood relatives such as spouses. According to Dr. Walter Gunn, 10–15% of PWCs have significant others with the illness (November 1991). Some researchers suspect that spouses and significant others of PWCs develop a greater risk over time of developing CFIDS due to increased viral "load," while others believe that the risk of contagion is high only in the early stages of the disease. And there is no evidence that CFIDS is contagious or transmissible. If CFIDS is indeed not highly contagious, genetic predisposition and/or exposure to environmental agents are more likely explanations of how the disease is contracted. Spouses and others close to the PWC may develop subclinical cases of CFIDS, according to Paul Cheney, M.D., Ph.D. (1991). In about 10% of cases in an outbreak in Lake Tahoe, both spouses became ill, and the risk of contagion to a spouse was highest in the first year of the illness. A parent and a child or children may fall ill at the same time. A study in Charlotte of patients with pets indicated that 50% of these pets were ill; this study has not been replicated and its significance is unknown. Because of the uncertainties regarding contagion, PWCs are advised not to be blood or organ donors. Some experts believe that PWCs should not obtain immunizations as these may challenge an already-disrupted immune process; others assert that flu shots pose no danger and are advisable. Because the transmissibility of the illness has not been determined, some physicians advise against anything that would cause con-tact with the saliva of the PWC, such as sharing eating utensils and drinking glasses or kissing on the mouth, and recommend the use of condoms for those who are sexually active with more than one partner. Other physicians feel that such precautions are unnecessary, so it is up to the individual to decide how cautious to be.

Although there is no known cure, CFIDS is treatable. Rest and lifestyle modification are the most helpful treatments. Active, driven, and highly-educated people may be more prone to CFIDS than their laid-back counterparts, and moderation in their activity levels falls somewhere between inconvenient and impossible. However, it is absolutely necessary to adapt by altering one's activity level. The worst thing PWCs can do is to go until they drop, thereby inviting relapses and possibly pro-longing the course of the illness. In addition to rest and moderation of activity, general and symptomatic treatments are available. It is essential to work with a physician who is knowledgeable about CFIDS and current treatment regimens. Individual and/or group psychotherapy are helpful for dealing with the emotional devas-tation that invariably accompanies CFIDS: illness-imposed limitations, anger, losses, depression, relationship and family issues, lifestyle alterations, and instruction in relaxation and stress-reduction techniques. Most support groups have referral lists of recommended professionals.

Is there life after CFIDS? *Do* people recover? About two-thirds of PWCs improve to the 80% or 90% level over a period of two to five years or more (Peterson, May 7, 1991) but some remain quite ill. Most who are able to resume a normal lifestyle find that they relapse during periods of intense stress or activity. Although many patients remain ill long-term, it is rare for the illness to become worse over time. It is impossible to predict which PWCs will recover, to what degree they will recover, or how long the illness will last in individual cases.

PWCs are encouraged to play an active role in treatment and to obtain current, accurate information. Appendix A contains numerous sources of information: publications and organizations that offer information about CFIDS treatment, research, patient advocacy, coping tips, and emotional support.

Although CFIDS continues to be the "unwanted stepchild of medicine" (in the words of Jay Goldstein, M.D.), the terms "yuppie flu" and "the malaise of the 80s" have fallen into disuse as the medical profession and the media now take a more serious approach to this devastating syndrome. There is no longer any question whether CFIDS is an organic illness. For PWCs and their significant others, it is only too real. Although they have fallen through the cracks of medicine, PWCs now expect to be taken seriously and treated appropriately. Although the CFIDS phenomenon remains inconvenient for and unpopular with patients, the medical profession, government agencies, and our society for numerous reasons, we must address CFIDS-related issues at all levels. We have no other choice.

PWCs have cause for hope. The medical community is becoming increasingly sensitive to CFIDS and those it afflicts; researchers are searching for causes, treatments, and cures; and a significant number of patients do recover—fully, or to some degree. Meanwhile, self-care, education, medical treatment, and emotional support remain the most precious resources of persons with CFIDS.

Chapter 2

◆

Definition and History of CFIDS

"Some doctors still dismiss its existence, but chronic fatigue syndrome could be the next crippling, global epidemic."

Marilee Strong
Mainstay: For the Well Spouse of the Chronically Ill

CFIDS: WHAT IT IS AND WHAT IT ISN'T

What CFIDS is ...

"CFIDS is a mystery waiting for a miracle," wrote one PWC. "CFIDS changes your priorities and puts you firmly in the *now*. You can't remember yesterday, and you can't predict tomorrow. When your *now* is full of pain and frustration, it's the end of the world. When your *now* improves, there's hope in your heart." CFIDS has been defined and described by many experts. Paul Cheney, M.D., noted that although we lack a specific definition of this syndrome, "we know it when we see it" (February 1990). He described the common denominator of PWCs as immune system dysregulation. Noting both similarities and differences among PWCs, Mark Loveless, M.D., calls CFIDS a "spectrum of disease."

Jay Goldstein, M.D., has referred to CFIDS as "the most complex disease I have ever studied." He defined CFIDS in March 1991: "I regard CFIDS as the final common pathway of a multifactorial psychoneuroimmunologic disorder with a limbic encephalopathy causing autonomic dysfunction and subtle neuroendocrine derangements." Although this definition is the most specific to date, it is difficult for those outside the medical profession to understand. Its essence is that disruption in normal brain functioning is the cause of most or all CFIDS symptoms, although the cause of the brain abnormalities are not currently known. Defining CFIDS as a psychoneuroimmunologic disorder encompasses all its systemic effects.

There may be a link between CFIDS and other illnesses. A study to compare CFIDS and multiple sclerosis is currently under way. A higher incidence of such disorders as endometriosis and interstitial cystitis (a type of bladder inflammation) is believed to exist among PWCs. (Other abnormalities found in PWCs are discussed in Chapters 4 and 5.)

Whether CFIDS patients are more or less likely than the healthy population to develop malignancies is unknown; some experts predict an increased risk and others a decreased risk of developing cancer. At present, no definite link between CFIDS and cancer has been established. One study indicated that healthy spouses of CFIDS patients may develop CFIDS-related abnormalities and possibly malignancies over time, but this study has not been replicated so the risk to spouses who are well is not known. Possible connections between CFIDS and malignancies are currently being studied.

One point of contention is whether CFIDS and fibromyalgia (FM) are separate, related, or identical illnesses. Although the FM label is most likely to be applied by rheumatologists, who see the patients most affected by joint and muscle pain, the consensus is that the two illnesses are much the same. The FM diagnosis is more common when pain is the prevalent symptom and when trigger and tender points are identified in the diagnostic process. (Such an examination is generally not made when pain is not the patient's primary complaint.) The similarities between the two diagnoses were explored and discussed at length at the First International CFS/FM Symposium in Los Angeles in 1990, and in several newsletter and journal articles, and if the two illnesses are not identical, they are certainly very closely related in terms of symptoms and certain measured abnormalities. Some researchers refer to FM as the myalgic form of CFIDS, others view FM as a symptom that is present in CFIDS and other illnesses such as lupus and arthritis. The incidence of fibromyalgia in the United States is high—an estimated six million patients. If the two illnesses come to be regarded as identical, the number of CFIDS/FM patients will be very high indeed.

We can only estimate the actual number of PWCs. Excluding those diagnosed with FM, estimates for CFIDS range from 2–10 million Americans, many of whom remain undiagnosed, with millions of additional cases in the United Kingdom, Australia, New Zealand, South Africa, and other countries. Although experts have developed these data, there is presently no reliable method for an accurate determination of the number of PWCs. But there are many more of us than anyone would have guessed just a few years ago! The research of Andrew Lloyd, M.D., suggests that there are 30–40 CFIDS cases per every 100,000 individuals in the general population (November 1991). One reason for the large number of undiagnosed patients is the lack of credibility afforded CFIDS and the general and inaccurate name used by the CDC and others (chronic fatigue syndrome). There are apparent "pockets" of CFIDS—areas in which a larger-than-normal percentage of cases develop—such as Incline Village, Nevada; New York; New Jersey; North Carolina; the Los Angeles area; and the San Francisco Bay Area. AIDS is also prevalent in some of these areas but the reason, if any, for the overlap is unknown. Unfortunately, the Centers for Disease Control surveillance effort to determine the number of CFIDS cases is confined to four cities that are not believed to be "hot spots." The number of CFIDS-related calls received by the CDC is estimated at 1–2,000 per month, and additional funding has been necessary to handle the large number of inquiries. Clearly this is an epidemic of huge proportions.

And what CFIDS isn't . . .

CFIDS isn't just chronic fatigue. The medical profession and general public have tended to confuse chronic fatigue and chronic fatigue syndrome, an unfortunate by-product of the terminology used for this illness. The name CFIDS is often preferred because it includes the "immune dysfunction" aspect of the illness, but the term CFS remains more widely used. The CDC insists on using this name, a point of contention for many researchers, practitioners, and PWCs.

CFIDS isn't "just" depression. Because fatigue is a symptom of depression, and because depression is a part of the CFIDS symptom complex, the distinction frequently becomes blurred. A recent article in a medical journal declared that chronic fatigue was simply a by-product of depression, making the misleading implication that the same was true for chronic fatigue syndrome. A retraction was later issued to correct the misleading notion that chronic fatigue *syndrome* was synonymous with depression. In most cases the onset of depression in PWCs occurs after the onset of CFIDS and is an effect rather than a cause of the syndrome. Chapter 4 contains a more detailed discussion of the clinical differences between CFIDS and depression.

CFIDS isn't AIDS. Viral involvement is common to both illnesses (evidence of activation or reactivation of such viruses as Epstein-Barr virus, cytomegalovirus, and human herpesvirus 6). Although the causal agent of AIDS is the human immunodeficiency virus (HIV), the causal role of a virus in CFIDS is suspected but has not been established, although non-HIV retroviruses are causal suspects.

With HIV disease the immune system is down-regulated, resulting in an immunocompromised state in which one is susceptible to opportunistic illnesses and infections. AIDS is fatal in most or all cases, whereas CFIDS tends to improve over time. Although some CFIDS-related deaths have been reported, this is a fairly unusual occurrence, and most have been suicides. As several PWCs have said, "The difference between AIDS and CFIDS is that AIDS kills you and CFIDS makes you wish you were dead."

In contrast to HIV diseases, CFIDS patients have dysregulated immune systems that are inappropriately "up-regulated"—as if an *on* switch had been pushed mistakenly—alternating with periods of "down-regulation." During the periods of down-regulation PWCs develop various infections such as upper respiratory infections and reactivation of other viruses. According to David Bell, M.D., the "degree of immune activation may be more severe in CFIDS, but the degree of immune deficiency is less severe" (1991, p. 13).

Other distinctions between the two diseases exist. Weight loss is associated with HIV disease, whereas weight gain is more common in CFIDS. Although the mode of transmission of CFIDS is unknown (it may be contagious only in its early stages—and even then only among those genetically predisposed), we know AIDS to be transmitted by bodily fluids such as blood, semen, and vaginal secretions. AIDS is considered a sexually transmitted disease, but there is no evidence that CFIDS is sexually transmitted. Although those with AIDS may be unusually susceptible to contracting CFIDS, the reverse is not true.

Still, similarities exist. Early AIDS, or ARC (AIDS-Related Complex), shares certain symptoms with CFIDS, and both follow a waxing and waning pattern. Incidence of activation or reactivation of other viruses is common to both. Both are currently considered epidemics posing serious health threats worldwide, and both have been insulted and ignored by the press, the medical profession, and government agencies.

The prejudices attached to both illnesses are based on myths—AIDS is no more a "gay disease" than CFIDS is "yuppie flu" or "crazy and lazy disease"—but such stigmas are widespread. However, AIDS research may ultimately be of great benefit to PWCs in that certain AIDS medications are helpful in treating CFIDS, and the causal viruses may indeed be related. Marc Iverson and Caryn Freese wrote in an excellent article about CFIDS and AIDS, "AIDS may be the disorder from which we can learn the most about CFIDS." (*The CFIDS Chronicle*, Spring/Summer 1990). But although the similarities between the two illnesses are eerie, CFIDS and AIDS are distinct entities.

A BRIEF HISTORY OF CFIDS

Outbreaks of CFIDS-like illnesses have been occurring in numerous countries including the United States for hundreds of years. The documented outbreaks have generally appeared in cooler countries rather than those with tropical climates: England, Scotland, Canada, Switzerland, Japan, Iceland, Australia, New Zealand, Germany, and South Africa. Outbreaks were given various names, including postviral fatigue syndrome, the English sweats, muscular rheumatism, neurasthenia, severe chronic active Epstein-Barr infection, chronic mononucleosis-like syndrome, Royal Free disease, Icelandic disease, postinfectious (or epidemic) neuromyasthenia, Addington's disease, vegetative neuritis, Akureyri disease, chronic hyper-fatigability syndrome, and benign myalgic encephalomyelitis (ME).

Unfortunately, these epidemics were only briefly noted in the medical literature and later forgotten. The similarities and possible connections among them have not been explored until relatively recently, when the incidence of numerous pocket epidemics finally received serious attention from the medical profession, government agencies, and the media. This attention was generated in large part by a grassroots movement among patients who were sick and tired . . . and sick and tired of not being taken seriously.

The current epidemic was first noted in Incline Village, Nevada, where a large portion of the population was stricken with an unusual illness in about 1984. Drs. Daniel Peterson and Paul Cheney treated many of these patients and in 1985 called upon the Centers for Disease Control (CDC) to investigate the outbreak, which occurred in surrounding areas as well. The CDC (Gary P. Holmes, M.D., and colleagues) initially denied the existence of an epidemic, but later claimed they had indeed taken it seriously and suspected it to be an Epstein-Barr-virus-related illness. Later the CDC retracted this stance, taking the position that the illness was real but was not likely caused by the Epstein-Barr virus, since tests indicated the presence of various other viruses as well which may or may not have played a causal role. The CDC, obviously uncomfortable and/or uninterested in this difficult syndrome, essentially turned its back on the devastation that was occurring not only in Incline Village but elsewhere. Stephen E. Straus, M.D., of the National Institute of Allergy and Infectious Diseases investigated the outbreak of CFIDS as well, taking the approach that since an etiologic agent (cause) hadn't been found, the illness may be a psychoneurotic disorder. Speaking and writing in double messages, Straus has acted both sympathetically and dubiously toward the CFIDS population, apparently concluding that psychopathology precedes the illness and is its primary cause. This concept does not fit with the majority of findings regarding CFIDS as a primarily organic disease. After consistent prodding, the CDC has become involved in researching CFIDS (or CFS, as they prefer to call it) but its efforts to date have been woefully inadequate—certainly disproportionate to the high incidence and devastation of CFIDS.

THE CFIDS PHENOMENON: STILL A MYSTERY

CFIDS has significantly affected us individually and collectively. In afflicting those in their most productive years, CFIDS is a serious threat to the nation's work force. The loss of workers, the mounting medical and research expenses, and the increasing number of disability cases and cumulative disability payments from Social Security and private insurers are potentially devastating to our national economy.

Also devastating are the divorce rate and suicide rate of PWCs. The divorce rate for chronically ill persons is an astounding 75%, and the suicide rate is unknown but believed to be high—perhaps six times that of the general population according to Hugh Fudenberg, M.D. (February 1990). Because many PWCs (including children and adolescents) feel overwhelmed, misunderstood, depressed, and hopeless, suicide becomes an strong option for a segment of the CFIDS population. Local and national CFIDS associations report large numbers of calls from suicidal patients but cannot estimate the number of patients who follow through and take their own lives.

Anthony Komaroff, M.D., wrote, "Chronic fatigue syndrome and its related conditions represent an illness distinct from other known physical and psychological illnesses," citing sudden onset, associated symptoms, and abnormalities found in PWCs (1988). Other researchers concur and are similarly baffled by this illness, which resembles other illnesses but is a phenomenon all its own. CFIDS is a disease like no other.

Chapter 3

◆

The Onset of CFIDS

SUDDEN ONSET OF A CHRONIC ILLNESS is unusual, but CFIDS is an exception. As one formerly active and healthy PWC says, "One day I got sick with what I assumed was the flu, but I never recovered." Abrupt onset of CFIDS in adults occurs in 75–90% of cases, often following a physically and/or emotionally traumatic event such as surgery, another illness, an accident or injury, vaccination, or a series of stressful incidents. Most common is onset with a flu-like illness, with neurological symptoms developing over time.

Others who develop CFIDS have a lifetime history of various illnesses, such as allergies, asthma, viral illnesses, PMS, irritable bowel syndrome, endometriosis, and bacterial infections. They become considerably sicker and begin to develop the markers of CFIDS, often over a period of time. Those in this category are often unable to pinpoint the onset of CFIDS because they have been ill so frequently. In fact, CFIDS may have actually been a factor in some of the earlier illnesses. Which came first—the illnesses or the CFIDS? The distinction is difficult to make, like the old "chicken or the egg" puzzle. Many patients who claimed to have been healthy all their lives have later realized that they were prone to various illnesses earlier in their lives but just shrugged them off, continued to work, and managed to function quite well. However, the sleep disorders, emotional problems (anxiety, depression, and mood swings), and various other neurological complaints were not commonly experienced prior to the onset of CFIDS.

Kyle describes retrospective confusion about her illness. "I may have been sick for five years and not really known it. I [had been] sick with pneumonia, depression, inability to concentrate. [Later on] I had every kind of blood test in the world and x-rays. I still didn't know what was wrong with me."

Patients who experience an abrupt onset of symptoms generally assume they have a "normal" or self-limiting illness that will linger for a week or two. Very few expect that this is the beginning of a long-term illness whose symptoms will wax and wane over time, and for which adequate treatment is difficult to obtain. Typically, patients begin to seek medical attention because their symptoms linger and because the symptom combinations and changes are so unusual. If the symptoms have not persisted for longer than a few weeks or months, a diagnosis of CFIDS is not usually made. Patients may be given appropriate medical treatment, including recommendations for rest, symptomatic treatment, and encouragement to obtain follow-up treatment if symptoms are not resolved within a given time frame. Patients who receive inappropriate medical attention do not feel their complaints are taken seriously and are generally told such things as "This is all in your head. You've just worn yourself out. Relax. Get a little rest and go back to work." Such reactions have been described repeatedly by patients who were frustrated with how awful they felt and how insensitively their physicians responded.

Some are fortunate enough to see physicians who take their complaints seriously, believing that the symptoms are real although the diagnosis is elusive. These physicians may say, "I don't know what you have, but let's find out," or "I think you may have CFS/CFIDS, but I really don't know much about it," followed by an appropriate referral. Most important at the outset is being taken seriously and treated respectfully.

As the symptoms linger for weeks and months, patients often experience a sense of unreality. Certain phrases are typical among prediagnosed PWCs: "What could be wrong with me? Why don't I get better? Why can't someone tell me what I have and just cure me? This can't be happening to me." Describing the onset of CFIDS, one PWC commented, "For no apparent reason, my life fell flat on its face."

I was not alarmed when I initially became ill—just tired, wiped out. This state of being was "not okay" for an active psychotherapist, college instructor, single mother, and exercise nut. I fought *it* hard, and *it* fought back harder. I experienced uncharacteristic mood swings, disequilibrium, and other bizarre symptoms. As additional symptoms developed, I sought medical advice and was told such nonsense as "You're too stressed. You need to exercise." (I had been a three-mile-a-day jogger, stopping only because jogging made me feel sicker—much, much sicker. When I explained this to my doc, he didn't seem to hear me.) "You're dehydrated. You're anxious." I was living in the Twilight Zone: my body had been hijacked by aliens and was doing mysterious things, not behaving like *my* body at all. And was I dehydrated? Anxious? Stressed? Maybe—but mainly I was vulnerable and confused. I couldn't trust my own perceptions and desperately needed information and understanding. I didn't get either.

Many PWCs formerly thrived on hectic lifestyles, striving for lives of perfection: the perfect student, employee, spouse, friend, parent. When CFIDS struck, these illusions crumbled as their optimism was replaced with a chaotic state of uncertainty, confusion, and fear.

Paula, a PWC, describes her experience:

When I first came down with it, I couldn't cope with anything. I wasn't working that hard at the time; I babysat and watched ten kids, all preschoolers, and I was taking a few classes. I couldn't function, I couldn't think clearly, and I was having a hard time with my studies, [I had difficulty] understanding the few simple courses I was taking. They weren't even difficult. I couldn't keep track of the bills to pay them. Little things . . . I'd go into a room and forget what I was going in there for and turn around and walk out again. I'd forget to call people back. I was snapping at everyone. Real dramatic. I couldn't cope. I'd cry very easily. I had physical and mental symptoms, and the confusion and frustration of trying to figure out what was wrong. At first I thought it was the flu and it would go away, but it didn't go away. I was fine one day and not fine the next—just that quick.

Notice Paula's comment: "I *wasn't working that hard* at the time"—a prime example of the self-imposed, unrealistically high standards of performance common to so many PWCs. Attending school and providing daycare for ten children *is* hard work, but such a high activity level was normal for Paula. Several patients and doctors have commented that even PWCs who cut back considerably on their activities are still busier than many of their healthy counterparts.

Bill, another PWC, describes the abrupt onset of CFIDS on Thanksgiving Day, November 1986, at the airport.

I was eating breakfast and I felt sick, like the flu came on. I can remember it very distinctly; it was as if a switch had been turned on. The onset was abrupt. The ride was a little tough; I felt weak—an "I need to get to bed" type of feeling, like a bad flu. The next thing I can remember was the pictures that were taken of me at the Thanksgiving dinner when I was bent over and my head was supported by one of my arms and I was really wiped out and sick. During that ten-day stay at my in-laws' house, I spent forty to sixty percent of the time in bed trying to sleep it off. I never really got better.

Yolanda, a recently remarried mother of three children, was attending law school when unusual symptoms began to appear. Her fatigue interfered with schooling and parenting, but she persevered and her symptoms increased in severity. She found that anything requiring mental activity made her sicker. She reported a "whole breakdown of my physical system," beginning with an ear infection and developing into "equilibrium and anxiety symptoms, numbness, shakiness, exhaustion, insomnia, allergic and viral-type problems." These problems developed and worsened over a period of several years, but Yolanda chose not to take the leave of absence from law school sug-

gested by her doctor. Then, as she began a review course for the
bar exam . . .

> I totally fell apart. My mind had to focus on a whole lot of
> material crammed into a short period of time. After a few
> weeks, I couldn't even stay alert. I felt paralyzed and would
> completely collapse. I would fall asleep and be in another
> zone; it was almost like passing out. I was just in a fog. I got
> really concerned, like maybe I had AIDS or something. It was
> really scary. Sometimes I'd feel fine, but within forty minutes
> of going to class, that was it; it was over. I thought maybe this
> was a psychological thing; 'I don't want to do this' or some-
> thing. It wasn't a fun thing to do, but I'd done a lot of other
> things that weren't fun, and I didn't pass out doing them.

Lack of family support made the ordeal worse. No one could
believe that "Superwoman" was having serious health problems.

In cases of acute onset, occasionally so severe as to require
hospitalization, the illness is regarded as more "real" and is
easier to diagnose. When the onset is gradual, bizarre symptoms
may take turns driving us crazy, while we're not "ill" enough for
it to be taken seriously by others. Then the diagnostic process
may take years. During those years of waiting to be labeled, the
illness may seem to disappear and reappear unpredictably.

In her book *Living with Chronic Illness*, Cheri Register writes
about the features of the initial phase of chronic illness, noting
the waxing and waning of symptoms, attempts to attribute
these symptoms to a psychological cause, difficulty obtaining a
diagnosis, and determination to chase the illness away by changing habits and behavior. She describes numerous frustrating
contacts with medical professionals as she sought the relief of
obtaining a specific diagnosis, compounded by strained relationships with others, continuous stress, and changes in mood
and personality.

Fear often accompanies the onset of strange, unexplained
symptoms. People wonder if they're going crazy, and not uncom-
monly fear they will die of whatever it is that has taken them
over. One patient comments: "I wondered if this is a terminal

thing, because I felt so tired and drained and burned out and couldn't manage to keep going like that. I figured it was going to kill me, whatever it was." And another: "I just couldn't go anymore. That wasn't like me. I could always say, 'I'm going to do this' and do whatever was necessary. My body didn't work right; I was scared, and I burst into tears. I was crying because I'm scared; I don't know what's going on." A common thread is the feeling of being out of control, captive of an unknown, invisible force that seemed to come out of nowhere.

Experiencing such symptoms is a frightening experience for anyone, especially when a diagnosis is not easily found. It feels terribly unfair that something alien, something beyond one's control can simply appear and change one's entire life. The onset of physical and emotional symptoms is accompanied by a reaction that generally includes disbelief, sorrow, and fear. The symptoms and accompanying emotional devastation continue interminably as the illness lingers.

Chapter 4

◆

Diagnosis:
The Search for a Label

Patient: Doc, I sure hope I'm sick!
Doctor: Why on earth would you wish that?
Patient: I'd sure hate to feel this awful if I were well!

THE NEED TO KNOW

We all know what it's like to feel well and what it's like to feel sick, but the distinction is difficult to put into words. I know I'm sick when I don't want to do the things that are normally pleasurable: not only do I feel physically unable, I don't even have the energy or interest to want to do those things. Such feelings are likely to be dismissed as merely emotional (i.e., crazy). To make matters worse, the symptoms of which I complain are often not observable or measurable, for example, joint pain, nausea, headache, light-headedness. And the symptoms come and go on their own schedule, inconveniencing and torturing me without permission or warning. Others have difficulty understanding how sick (how absolutely rotten) we feel, in part because our numerous symptoms are invisible. "You look fine," they tell us. "You look mah-velous!" It is *not* better to look good than to feel good!

25

Our society has many rules about being ill, most of them unwritten. In general, people who become ill are expected to do one of two things: recover or die. It's okay to break a limb—as long as it heals in a timely manner and one does not complain excessively. Even an occasional headache, which is invisible, is acceptable and easily remedied. But to have symptoms that cannot be seen or understood by others is not okay. Anything that cannot be either fixed or denied makes trouble.

The PWC has an especially hard time "legitimizing" the illness. Sometimes a diagnosis is made fairly quickly, but in many cases years elapse between onset and diagnosis. Often the individual symptoms are not cause for alarm, but the number of symptoms experienced and the length of time they persist are problematic. The symptoms vary so much that it can take some time before it becomes apparent that they are all part of one syndrome. Patients experiencing facial numbness, for example, may not mention such a trivial, seemingly irrelevant symptom to their doctors but will respond positively if asked whether they have experienced such a symptom. Often patients feel they can ignore the minor symptoms, assuming them to be transient. Many patients have seen doctors who did not take their complaints seriously, and so have given up the pursuit of a diagnosis. Still others feel crazy reporting the numbers of varied symptoms they are experiencing; to visit a doctor complaining of depression, fatigue, equilibrium problems, brain fog, sore joints, shortness of breath, headache, ringing in the ears, and on and on . . . . Sounds pretty crazy, doesn't it? An approach-avoidance issue emerges: "I want a diagnosis, but I don't want to have to recite that crazy list of symptoms again and risk being told what I am secretly beginning to suspect—that I'm bonkers. I'm not handling my life right; I'm not coping; I'm copping out—can't take the strain, not bearing up; I'm crazy and lazy. I'm afraid it might be true, even though I *know* this is organic, a virus or something . . . . There's something chewing on my wiring, sabotaging the controls. I'm not making this up; I'm really ill, really I am. You've got to believe me, doctor, even though if I were you, I probably wouldn't believe me, either. What is *happening* to me?"

The patient needs to be listened to and taken seriously. PWCs do not enjoy being ill, nor do they have anything to gain by pretending they are. It's easier, however, for society to dismiss those who have chronic complaints, who feel lousy much of the time, as people who just don't want to participate. We don't follow the rules. We slip through the cracks. We may not be well enough to go to work but may not be ill enough to spend all our time in bed. Some days we can accomplish a lot, other days mere survival needs require all of our limited energy. We are not an easy lot to deal with. Ask any doctor or family member of a PWC. For no apparent reason, our bodies and minds are not behaving themselves. We want—*need*—some sort of explanation for this. We want to know why and what to do about it. In the beginning we'll settle for a label, anything that validates our experience and reassures us we're not nuts.

Step One in the diagnostic process is to schedule an appointment with a doctor. The receptionist generally wants to know what the problem is, but usually the description of one's malady is so lengthy it will be interrupted several times by other incoming calls. The appointment may be granted as if it were a special favor rather than a two-way business transaction, and the preparation begins. "What can I say so the doctor will understand the seriousness of this; how can I describe what is happening to me? If I bring a list, the doc will think I'm neurotic. If I don't, I'm likely to forget a lot of important information. How healthy should I look? If I look okay, I won't be taken seriously. But what can I do? Paint circles under my eyes? Draw red dots all over my body? I know I'm sick, so why should it be so difficult to convince someone else? And why should I have to convince anyone?"

As Sefra Pitzele wrote, we are in a "well until proven sick" situation. Although she is afflicted with lupus rather than CFIDS, her experiences will sound familiar to PWCs. She describes the unexpected rush of exhaustion that defies any standard definition of fatigue, the accompanying feelings of helplessness, and the search for a diagnosis. During this time we continually hear that our doctors cannot find any specific problem, and self-doubt sets in as we wonder if our symptoms are imagined or fabricated. "As our confidence in our own judgment erodes still further, we depend more and more on the judgment of those people who seem to have grown numb to our complaints. Before long, we don't know what to believe" (1985, p. 26). And we can even forget what it felt like to be well.

Bill says of his quest for a diagnosis:

> There were periods where I would have probably accepted any diagnosis just to get a diagnosis, but I'm to the point where I'm glad I don't have what they've been testing me for, even though it's driving me nuts and I'm feeling lousy and I still don't know if I'm going to be alive or what the hell's going on with me. It's frustrating. You don't really want to hear that you've got something that's going to kill you so that people will believe you're sick!

At our wits' end and with self-esteem at low ebb, we are surrounded by others who cannot understand how we feel. Armchair advice and diagnoses from concerned others may do more harm than good, and the same is true of the reactions of many of the doctors we approach with desperation and fear. Still we pursue a diagnosis: proof that we are really ill, that our symptoms—and we ourselves—are legitimate.

DEALING WITH DOCTORS

There is some argument as to whether diagnosis is an art or a science; ideally, it is a skilled combination of both. The expertise and intuition of the diagnostician supplemented with diagnostic tests are likely to yield the most useful information.

I wonder, if I didn't have this illness but were a doctor listening to someone who did, what would I think? I'd like to think that I'd take a patient-oriented, caring approach. That I'd listen, taking the patient's words seriously, and be willing to say "I don't know" if I didn't know. I'd like to think I wouldn't cop out and that I'd keep an open mind.

Humorist Dave Barry describes the "two most popular doctor options: to tell you to come back in a week, or to send you to the hospital for tests. Another option would be to say, 'It sure beats the heck out of me why your tongue is swollen,' but that could be a violation of the Hippocratic Oath." He suggests that perhaps only conditions involving "say, an icepick protruding from your skull" are likely to elicit a conclusive diagnosis, and that in the case of subtler problems, "you may never find out what's wrong" (1988). His statements are humorous and exaggerated, but his point is valid: diagnosing an elusive illness can be exceptionally difficult, especially when the cause is unknown and no specific diagnostic tests have been developed. The process is perplexing for the medical profession as well as patients and their families.

Most patients see several doctors before a correct diagnosis of CFIDS is made. Many patients see five, ten, or fifteen doctors; an astounding number see even more. It takes determination to continue the search, and my hunch is that many give up along the way. Although the CFIDS awareness level of the medical profession has improved, many doctors still don't "believe in" chronic fatigue syndrome. But we're not talking about believing in ghosts or believing in God; we're talking about doctors believing their patients, their educated colleagues, and the medical literature. We are dealing with a serious problem and we need to work at finding out more about it rather than doubting those who have it.

Those who have had to search for a doctor who would take their reports seriously and work with them to find a cause have horror stories to tell about the process. Unfortunately, the fields of psychiatry and psychology become dumping grounds for those with elusive illnesses. When nothing "turns up" on lab tests, the patient is often presumed physically healthy but psychologically suspect.

Despite the psychological aspects of CFIDS, to assume that psychological factors cause the syndrome is to confuse correlation with causation. CFIDS generally occurs out of the blue, with a sudden onset and a host of physical symptoms that do not ordinarily accompany depression or anxiety syndromes —a fact often conveniently overlooked by those unwilling to delve into the unknown. The physician's personal feelings and judgment about the perceived mental status of the patient—as well as over-reliance on technology to provide definitive answers —can result in incorrect, often damaging, conclusions.

I saw a family practitioner, an otolaryngologist, a neurologist, a gynecologist, a gastroenterologist, an allergist, a cardiologist, and a host of other -ologists before finding out what might be wrong. I could write pages about the expense, self-doubt, emotional turmoil, degradation, and confusion I experienced. I got angry alternately at the doctors and at myself. Many of them took my complaints seriously—those who had known me prior to the onset of my symptoms and didn't consider me a garden-variety "hysterical female." The doctors who hadn't known me B.C. (before CFIDS) more often treated me like a "crock," a neurotic woman with multisystem complaints who probably enjoyed being attended to by the medical profession. The process was agonizing. The illness itself was crazy-making; the insult added by insensitive, disbelieving physicians made the ordeal worse.

The anxiety of waiting for test results was more traumatic than the tests themselves. Like a teenager waiting to be asked to the prom, I sat near the telephone waiting to hear whether I had a brain tumor, hypoglycemia, heart problems, multiple sclerosis, an ulcer.... Initially I was relieved to know that I didn't have the dread disease of the week, then I became frightened again not to know what I *did* have. I assumed that if the right test were run, I'd have the information I needed and then could do whatever was indicated to get well. With each negative test result I became *more* rather than less concerned because of the implied conclusion that I didn't "have" anything at all. I had been taught to believe in the wisdom of doctors and medical tests, but felt misunderstood, mistreated, and mislabeled. I look back and shudder. Two incredibly long years went by before I was properly diagnosed by a competent and thorough physician.

Bill described the diagnostic crazies he experienced during all the testing and doctor visits:

I got more and more depressed and finally got to the point where I was totally devastated. I'd been through heart tests and neurological tests, I'd been to an infectious disease doctor, I'd been through blood tests time and time again. My family doctor thought I might have E-B virus . . . . Although some doctors don't believe in it, she says too many people are having those symptoms. She believes it exists; she's more into calling an apple an apple. So I got into thinking that's what I've got, and the infectious disease specialist says, "I don't think you've got a viral problem, but I don't know what it is." Everything else is ruled out, but this is one thing you can't rule out. That doesn't mean you can rule it in. It's another vague diagnosis.

I saw another doctor and told him half the doctors don't take me seriously. He said, "I'm taking you very seriously. We need to look at several areas, including allergy and immunology." He thinks what I've been through is a travesty.

Sometimes the doctor does everything she or he can think of and finds no cause. That is understandable; we are dealing with an elusive and ill-defined phenomenon. To be told, as Bill later was, "The truth of it, quite honestly, is that I don't know what the hell you have. I don't know what else to check. I don't think it's going to kill you," is at least an honest statement. But to be told, "I can't find anything, so it must be a psychological problem. Go see a shrink" is not a constructive or fair statement to make. An honest "I don't know" is acceptable, but placing blame on the patient is totally inappropriate. To do so reinforces the irrational notion that we are responsible for being ill. Bill later said, "A smart doctor . . . will tell you that he can't find what's wrong with you, not that you have a psychological problem. People can be really damaged by that kind of a physician."

In his recent book *What Your Doctor Didn't Learn in Medical School*, Stuart Berger wrote that many patients, particularly women, get stamped with the label "hypochondriac" or "hysteric" when it's unclear what's ailing them. Berger discussed the attitude of most doctors confronted with patients reporting vague symptoms who just don't feel like themselves anymore. Doctors often become annoyed and skeptical because they are not well-acquainted with some of the more elusive illnesses. Many times the symptoms are diverse and vague, the clues are subtle, and the search is frustrating.

However, when a physician has seen a number of CFIDS patients, the picture becomes clearer to them. Byron Hyde, M.D., said, "This is a simple disease to diagnose despite what you've heard to the contrary. There is no disease even vaguely like it" (February 1990).

THE PROCESS OF DIAGNOSIS

The diagnostic criteria for Chronic Fatigue Syndrome were defined in a landmark article that appeared in the March 1988 *Annals of Internal Medicine*. This article was coauthored by physicians from the Centers for Disease Control and several prominent CFIDS researchers. Its authors described "a combination of nonspecific symptoms . . . with a remarkable absence of objective physical or laboratory abnormalities" (p. 387). The authors criticized the common practice among physicians of basing a diagnosis of CFIDS solely on EBV antibody titer test results. Their stated purpose in developing a case definition was to allow systematic further study of the illness. They have based the diagnostic criteria on symptoms (problems reported by the patient), signs (those that the physician can measure), duration, degree of impairment, and the ruling out of other disorders with similar symptoms. The authors emphasized that this illness is a "syndrome" (a complex of symptoms occurring together) and may not be a discrete disease entity. There may be multiple causes for this group of symptoms. Unfortunately, this definition excludes many patients who have the illness but do not exactly meet the criteria, which are limited in scope. Numerous researchers have recommended using a new set of diagnostic criteria or at least adding to the symptom criteria in this definition, but the CDC is currently holding to this narrow definition of CFIDS. For example, those with depression and other psychological/psychiatric disorders are excluded from the patient population according to this strict definition—and virtually every PWC experiences such problems as a part of the illness! Additionally, people with prior psychiatric problems may develop CFIDS just as anyone else could, but they are excluded from the case definition. I doubt there are any other conditions that exclude those with previously diagnosed psychological problems. The physician may make a clinical diagnosis of CFIDS even if an individual case does not meet the strict CDC research criteria.

The CDC definition underemphasizes the numerous signs of neurological impairment—hallmarks of CFIDS—in its definition. Several CFIDS experts have stated the belief that this definition _excludes_ more PWCs than it _includes_! Numerous additional symptoms associated with CFIDS are listed and described in Chapter 5. These criteria need to be revised to reflect the most significant symptoms and recently discovered abnormalities.

Symptom criteria as listed in the primarily CDC-authored article are quite specific. For a positive diagnosis, both Major Criteria 1 and 2 must be satisfied, as well as at least eight of the eleven symptom criteria, or at least six of the eleven symptom criteria and at least two of the three physical criteria.

Major criteria (both must be met)

1. "New onset of persistent or relapsing, debilitating fatigue or easy fatigability in a person who has no previous history of similar symptoms, that does not resolve with bedrest, and that is severe enough to reduce or impair average daily activity below 50% of the patient's premorbid [pre-illness] activity level for a period of at least six months" (p. 388).

2. Exclusion of other clinical conditions that may produce the same or similar symptoms.

Minor criteria

Symptom criteria (eight must be met): These symptoms must have begun during or after the onset of increased fatigue and must have persisted or recurred over a period of six months or more. All symptoms do not have to have occurred simultaneously.

1. Mild fever or chills

2. Sore throat

3. Painful lymph nodes

4. General muscle weakness

5. Muscle discomfort or pain

6. Prolonged (more than 24 hours) fatigue following exercise that would have been easily tolerated prior to onset of illness

7. Headaches (different type or severity than those experienced prior to onset of symptoms)

8. Arthralgia (aching joints) without swelling or redness

9. Neurophysiological complaints (at least one: sensitivity to light, visual problems, forgetfulness, irritability, confusion, difficulty thinking or concentrating, depression)

10. Sleep disturbance (excessive sleep or inability to sleep)

11. Onset of this cluster of symptoms occurring over a brief period of time, such as a few hours or a few days.

Or six of the above minor criteria *and* two of the following physical criteria must be met:

Physical criteria

1. Low-grade fever

2. Nonexudative pharyngitis [sore throat]

3. Tender or swollen lymph nodes, primarily in the neck or armpit.
(Holmes, Kaplan, Gantz, Komaroff, Schonberger, Straus, Jones, DuBois, Cunningham-Rundles, Pahwa, Tosato, Zegans, Purtilo, Brown, Schooley, & Brus, *Annals of Internal Medicine*, 1988)

David Bell, M.D., uses different criteria for diagnosis based on symptoms alone. He diagnoses CFIDS when symptoms have persisted for at least six months and when six of the eight "major symptoms" are present: fatigue, neurologic complaints, recurrent sore throat, lymphatic pain, muscle pain, joint pain, headache, and abdominal pain; or when five of these last symptoms plus two of the following are present: fever/chills/night sweats, eye pain/eye sensitivity, and skin rash. In addition, Dr. Bell has developed a different set of criteria for diagnosing CFIDS in children, which is described in Chapter 9 (1991, p. 35).

Most physicians who are knowledgeable about CFIDS agree that the patient's history and description of symptoms are more helpful than the physical examination because many of the reported symptoms and sensations cannot be felt or measured. Because there is no definitive test for CFIDS, the diagnosis is based upon the exclusion of illnesses with similar symptoms. This process can be lengthy, stressful, and expensive, but if there is another illness present, particularly one that is curable or treatable, such information is essential. The tendency to self-diagnose is natural, especially when one's symptoms match those described by friends or in the media, but it is important to have one's suspicions confirmed by a professional who is experienced in diagnosing CFIDS.

Illnesses to be ruled out vary from case to case based upon the patient's signs and symptoms. Syndromes with similar symptoms that should be ruled out include:

Other viral illnesses, such as
— cytomegalovirus (CMV)
— chronic mononucleosis (Epstein-Barr virus infection)
— toxoplasmosis
— herpesviruses (simplex I and II, herpes zoster, HHV-6)
— mycoplasmal pneumonia
— coxsackie-B
— hepatitis A and B, chronic active hepatitis
— rubella
— HIV (ARC/AIDS)

— HHV-6
— toxoplasmosis
Other infectious diseases, such as
— localized infections
— bacterial infections (e.g., tuberculosis, brucellosis,
    endocarditis, Lyme disease)
collagen vascular diseases (e.g., systemic lupus
    erythematosus)
rheumatoid arthritis
immune deficiency state (e.g., low Immunoglobin A,
    which helps fight infection)
chronic inflammatory diseases (e.g. sarcoidosis,
    Wegener's granulomatosis)
toxic agents (e.g., chemical solvents, heavy metals, and
    pesticides)
allergies
malignancies, especially lymphoma
chronic psychiatric diseases (e.g., depression, anxiety,
    and/or panic disorder as the sole cause of symptoms)
chronic systemic diseases (e.g., pulmonary, renal [kidney],
    cardiac, hepatic [liver], hematologic [blood]
anemia
neuromuscular diseases (e.g., multiple sclerosis and
    myasthenia gravis)
fungal diseases, including candidiasis (which may be a
    separate illness or part of the CFIDS cluster)
endocrine diseases such as hypothyroidism, Addison's
    disease, Cushing's syndrome, diabetes mellitus
parasitic infection (giardiasis, toxoplasmosis, amoebiasis,
    or helminthic infection)
drug side effects, dependency or abuse (including
    alcohol)
Drug interactions

Note: Evidence of viral infection may be an alternate diagnosis
or may be a CFIDS-related phenomenon. This is true of other
listed conditions as well.

LABORATORY TESTS

In my own quest for a diagnosis I consulted many doctors, some of whom dismissed my complaints as trivial, psychogenic, or illusory. Others listened to me carefully and made a genuine attempt to discover the cause of the abrupt changes in my life.

The lab test ordeal was emotionally and financially draining. The testing procedures themselves were fairly innocuous, inducing only moderate discomfort in the worst cases, whereas the cost of the tests produced great discomfort. Waiting for test results was the worst aspect of the process. Although my gut feeling was that I didn't have any of the frightening illnesses for which I was tested, I knew I had something I couldn't identify. The possibility that I had a degenerative, malignant, or terminal condition created anxious hours and days as I waited for results. My future husband and I had become involved prior to the onset of my illness. We had planned to marry but had not set a date. Following my recovery from a severe exacerbation (and a morning of diagnostic tests), we decided to celebrate by getting married that very afternoon. The EEG and a C-T scan added a more dramatic touch than the routine blood test of yore. The line about "in sickness and in health" in the wedding ceremony caused us to snicker (my mother cried), but I was truly concerned about my brand-new husband marrying a Typhoid Mary . . . or, in any case, someone with an unknown, undiagnosed, strange, life-altering illness. It was a memorable day for many reasons. The test results were negative.

Sophisticated laboratory tests can be of great value, but there are some dangers associated with their use. The emphasis on this aspect of diagnosis has been damned as well as praised, often by doctors themselves. In 1988, Andrew Weil, M.D., a Harvard-trained physician, wrote about the problems incurred by an increasing dependency on lab tests. He believes that with selective questioning and active listening on the part of the physician, the patient will in essence describe the diagnosis. Weil pointed out the danger of reliance on technology as a replacement for—rather than an adjunct to—the judgment of artful diagnosticians, as well as his concern that normalizing test results rather than treating patients becomes the goal of treatment.

Diagnostic tests are routine matters for the medical personnel who perform them, but the experience is quite different for the patient. These tests are journeys into unknown places, invasions of privacy, strange and often unexplained violations. Even when they are not painful, many tests evoke discomfort and anxiety. The patient's fears are generally not allayed or even addressed by those who perform the tests or those who impart the results.

In *The Healing Heart,* author Norman Cousins lamented the lack of human warmth in the performance of tests. Cousins wrote that the process is often detrimental to the patient and that the patient frequently feels diminished by the process. He cautioned that the hazards of the testing procedures themselves as well as the patient's induced fears should be considered. The equipment and procedures are frightening and intimidating, and technology can create panic.

We await test results as if they and not ourselves are the ultimate authority about our state of health. We place greater value on so-called scientific data than on intuition and judgment. And often the findings are not even standardized, since each lab sets its own standards for normalcy. Great variations often exist among the findings of different labs, and errors may be made for a number of reasons, resulting in false negative or false positive results.

In her account of her own quest for a diagnosis, Toni Jeffreys wrote in *The Mile-High Staircase* that the laboratory becomes the focus of the diagnostic process, with the actual patient playing only a minor role, appearing in "bits and pieces" or "fluids" that are tested. "And when there is a discrepancy between the laboratory and the patient, it has to be the patient who is inadequate, not the laboratory.... Without a positive test, there can be no diagnosis. Without a diagnosis, illness doesn't exist," wrote Jeffreys.

When test results are within normal limits, the temptation to label the patient a neurotic, somatizer, or malingerer is apparently strong. The barbaric, insulting, and often condescending practice of referring such "nut cases" or "crocks" to psychiatrists is a great blind spot in the practice of medicine and an affront to those with difficult-to-diagnose illnesses. The patient feels blamed for the illness, accused of an inability to cope with stress, an ineffective life adjustment, a desire for attention, or an enjoyment of being ill. It is too often forgotten that information provided by a laboratory must be regarded as only part of a larger picture, and that illness can exist in the absence of supporting laboratory data.

Although diagnosis of CFIDS is currently based on specific criteria rather than lab tests, such studies may offer useful information about the nature and treatment of CFIDS.

Specific tests

In order to assess the patient's status and rule out other disorders, certain lab tests should be performed. A basic diagnostic workup includes some the following tests as appropriate:

> Complete blood count
> SMA-20
> Sedimentation (sed) rate
> Tuberculin skin test and/or chest x-ray
> Urinalysis
> Thyroid profile
> Antinuclear antibody
> HIV
> Lyme disease
> Stool specimen test for parasites
> Viral antibodies (HHV-6, EBV, CMV, etc.)
> Exercise testing with oxygen consumption measurements
> Lupus panel
> Antithyroid antibodies
> Serum copper
> Neurological or neuropsychological tests
> Minnesota Multiphasic Personality Inventory (MMPI)
> Brain imaging, including magnetic resonance imaging (MRI), PET scan, BEAM scan, and NeuroSPECT scan (measures cerebral blood flow)

Functional capacity evaluation
Immune tests, including circulating immune complexes,
   IgA levels and IgG subclasses

More controversial tests include toxic chemical analysis, vestibular (balance) testing, and Single Lymphocyte Immune Function Test (SLIF). Additionally, the Karnofsky Performance Scale may be used to measure daily activities.

Abnormal results found on these tests may be used to diagnose CFIDS, determine appropriate treatment, and provide documentation for disability insurance purposes. In addition to the above tests, a detailed history as well as serial weight and temperature measurements offer relevant diagnostic information. A patient-kept calendar of symptom activity over time and the use of a symptom checklist are very helpful in the diagnostic process. (See the Symptom Checklist on p. 297.)

Measurement of Epstein-Barr antibody titers is not appropriate for diagnosing CFIDS. Most doctors and patients have found that the results of the EB antibody tests generally do not correlate with overall symptom severity. This test may have application, however, in determining treatment. EBV antibody titers vary among patients, and there is considerable variation among results obtained from different labs. The test is also quite expensive.

Special tests of immune and neurological functioning can be helpful in detecting abnormalities in CFIDS patients. Because findings have been inconsistent, it is not known if all CFIDS patients have the same types of dysfunction, or whether immune dysfunction is a cause or effect of the syndrome. There are many aspects of immune and neurological functioning we are not currently able to identify or measure.

The tests listed above help us to rule out other conditions. Some newly-developed tests may be of more help in ruling in CFIDS. One test called CARA (CFIDS Associated Retrovirus Assay) tests for certain markers for a certain viral agent. Other tests will likely be developed as a result of current research that will help us to pinpoint a diagnosis.

ABNORMALITIES

Various multisystem abnormalities have been detected in CFIDS patients, but findings are not consistent. The abnormalities vary widely among patients, but certain clusters of findings form patterns. Until testing is standardized we will not have a way of using the data to provide diagnostic certainties.

The following abnormalities have been noted by various researchers and presented at medical conferences and in medical literature:

> Immune Abnormalities: cytokine dysfunction (e.g., elevation of alpha interferon, elevation of interleukins 1 and 2), lymphocyte abnormalities, elevated herpes group virus antibodies (e.g., Epstein-Barr virus, CMV, HHV-6), altered T4/T8 ratio and T-cell activation and low T-cell counts, low natural killer (NK) cell numbers and function, ele-vated 2-5A synthetase and RNAse L, allergies, antinuclear antibodies, antithyroid antibodies, IgG (immunoglobin) deficiencies. (*Note:* Although abnormalities vary from one patient to another, impaired function of NK cells are one consistent finding, according to Anthony Komaroff, M.D., November 1991)
>
> Brain/Central Nervous System Abnormalities: lesions in certain parts of the brain, cerebral hypoperfusion (insufficient blood flow to certain parts of the brain—especially after exercise, when it would increase in healthy subjects), abnormal brain responses (as measured by N-1/P-1 complex), hypothalamic dysregulation, and altered brain metabolism, cognitive dysfunction, intellectual deficits, memory consolidation, spatial perception and organization, corticotropin releasing hormone (CRH) and cortisol level deficiencies
>
> Psychological/Neuropsychological Test Scores: decreased IQ scores, distinct pattern of scores on MMPI, poor

performance on certain memory tests, impaired
performance on neuropsychological subtests

Altered sleep patterns and sleep wave physiology

Recurrent infections, candidiasis, and parasitic infection

Low sedimentation rate: 0–3, with transient periods of
increase into the 30s–50s (normal is 0–20)

Blood studies: elevated or decreased (often fluctuating)
white blood cell count, (mild leukopenia, moderate
monocytosis, relative lymphocytosis, slightly elevated
SGOT and SGPT), high red blood cell count,
abnormal red cell membranes, elevation of serum
angiotensin-converting enzyme (ACE)

Low levels of zinc and magnesium

Low exercise capacity and oxygen consumption,
inefficient glucose usage in exercise; exaggerated
increase in blood pressure and erratic breathing
patterns during exercise

Neuromuscular abnormalities, including altered
metabolism in the muscles

Fever, low body temperatures

Low metabolic rate

Elevated liver enzymes

Alkaline urine

Endocrine dysfunction

Loss of ridging in the fingertips, causing loss of fingerprints.

(*Note:* This information is based on the work of Drs. Archard,
Bastien, Behan, Caliguiri, Cheney, Daly, DuBois, Findley, Fuden-
berg, Goldstein, Grufferman, Gupta, Handleman, Herberman, Hyde,
Iger, Jessop, Jones, Klimas, Komaroff, Landay, Levy, Lieberman,
Lloyd, Loblay, Lottenberg, Loveless, Mena, Moldofsky, Olson, Peter-
son, Rozofsky, Sandman, Suhadolnik, Tosato, Wakefield, and others.)

The more significant findings warrant further discussion. Immune
abnormalities are becoming more apparent as testing becomes
more sophisticated. Paul Cheney, M.D., uses a radial plot to
identify overall patterns, which are more helpful than individual measures. Many of the immune abnormalities suggest up-
regulation of the immune system. A recent discovery discussed

by Drs. Daniel Peterson and Paul Cheney is the natural immunity pathway, the intracellular process of the immune system that defends against cellular invasion and viral replication, in which 2-5A synthetase plays a vital part. When this function is disrupted, every cell of the body can be affected.

Brain scans reveal various abnormalities previously listed. These abnormalities manifest themselves throughout the body, resulting in multiple symptoms. Results of brain scans and neurological functioning indicate that certain parts of the brain are more impaired than others. In extensive neuropsychological testing of PWCs, Sheila Bastien, Ph.D., has found abnormal results on tests of memory, spatial organization, visual discrimination, sequencing problems, abstract reasoning, and IQ scores. Abnormalities were identified through the use of a battery of tests including Draw-A-Person, Wechsler Adult Intelligence Scale-Revised (WAIS-R), Wechsler Memory Scale, Knox Cubes, MMPI, and the Halstead-Reitan. The cluster of abnormalities is indicative of a multifocal pattern of impairment not found in other illnesses (November 1990; May 1991).

Scores on the MMPI form a unique profile unlike any seen in other disorders. This unique finding was made by Linda Miller Iger, Ph.D., (_The CFIDS Chronicle_, Spring/Summer 1990) and has been replicated. On the WAIS-R, Sheila Bastien, Ph.D., (May 1991) found significantly depressed IQ scores and lower-than-expected scores on certain subtests, including digit span and symbol (backwards only), picture completion, block design, and object assembly. IQ scores measured in children with CFIDS indicated different areas of impairment, and additional studies are in progress. Draw-A-Person test results revealed drawings with strong indicators of impairment. Overall, Bastien noted significant impairment in verbal recall, spatial perception, and motor functioning, and mild impairment in visual recall and abstract reasoning. Kurt Sandman, M.D., (May 1991) noted significant memory impairments, especially in terms of taking in and encoding (integrating and recording) new memories. He, too, found a unique profile of PWCs on neurometric tests and also found a correlation between scores on memory tests and immune abnormalities.

Assessment and comparison of lab test results are made more difficult by the fluctuation of these abnormalities over time. For more specific information readers are referred to Dr. Jay Goldstein's book *CFS: The Struggle for Health*, Dr. David Bell's book *The Disease of a Thousand Names*, the article "Immunologic Abnormalities in Chronic Fatigue Syndrome" (Klimas, et al.; see Bibliography), and articles in *The CFIDS Chronicle*.

At present there is no standard method of diagnosing CFIDS. A standardized testing sequence would be advantageous to the patient and facilitate more systematic data for researchers.

RULING OUT DEPRESSION

Although depression almost invariably accompanies CFIDS, it is not the cause of the illness. Common to both CFIDS and major depressive disorder (MDD) are fatigue, lethargy, anhedonia (inability to experience pleasure), sleep disruption, lowered activity level, impaired concentration and memory, decreased libido, and weight changes, but MDD shares only some of the features of CFIDS. Researchers at the National Institute of Health, however, are reluctant to dismiss the psychological angle, ignoring most clinical research and insisting that CFIDS is an illness of psychoneurotic origin. Unfortunately, many physicians cling to the "psychologized" notion of CFIDS, continuing to misdiagnose and mistreat their patients. As a side note, one physician in the Phoenix area has told me repeatedly that CFIDS does not exist, that what we are seeing are fatigued, depressed individuals in search of a new label. His college-age daughter has recently been diagnosed with this disease, which he has recently (and reluctantly) admitted is a real illness—although an extremely rare one!

In order to distinguish between depression and CFIDS as the primary cause of an individual's symptoms, the following differences should be noted.

1. Onset. CFIDS begins in a majority of patients with a flu-like illness, but acute onset is not characteristic of MDD. The vast majority of PWCs do not have a history of major depression. Although many PWCs experience depression (as do those with other chronic illnesses), some PWCs are not depressed. In many cases depression decreases later in the course of the illness.

2. Incidence. CFIDS occurs in both epidemic and endemic forms, that is, outbreaks occur but individuals may develop it any time. Depression has never been known to exist in epidemic form, but pockets or local outbreaks of CFIDS are common.

3. Major symptoms. The primary symptoms of depression are feelings of hopelessness and helplessness. The exaggerated feelings of guilt and the tendency to be overly self-critical that are characteristic of primary depression are not usually characteristic of CFIDS-related depression. Although such feelings are experienced by many PWCs, they are not the primary symptoms of the illness. Those with MDD generally do not wish to be active; most PWCs would like to be active but are physically unable. A depressed individual would not generally experience most of the physical and neurological deficits found in CFIDS: sore throat; tender or swollen lymph nodes; unusual headaches; body pain; nausea; irritable bowel syndrome-type symptoms; unusual sensitivities to medications, odors, and other substances; decreased blood flow to the brain following exercise; memory disturbances; photosensitivity; word-finding difficulty; visual discrimination and sequencing problems; altered spatial perception; abstract reasoning difficulties; aphasia and dyscalculia (difficulty using words and numbers); disequilibrium; etc. On various memory tests, PWCs perform poorly as compared to depressed patients and to healthy controls. Depressed patients exhibit slower motor speed than PWCs, who evidence decreased mental speed.

4. Laboratory test results. Immunological, neurological, and endocrine measures yield different results for the two disorders. Certain immune and neurological abnormalities found in CFIDS are not known to occur in MDD. Changes in cerebral perfusion (blood flow to parts of the brain) are significantly different in PWCs from those with major depression.

5. Response to treatment. Although the medications used to treat MDD are helpful to PWCs, they do not cause the type of overall improvement found in those who are depressed. In addition, the amount of antidepressant medication commonly administered to PWCs for symptom relief is extremely low as compared to dosages for those with MDD. (For example, Sinequan, a tricyclic antidepressant, is used by PWCs to improve sleep and decrease pain in dosages of 2–20 mg per day. In the treatment of depression, the initial dose of Sinequan would generally be 50 mg, increasing to 150 mg or more over time.) It is believed that certain antidepressants administered in doses much lower than those used for treating MDD create improvement in CFIDS by exerting immunomodulating properties, affecting certain neurotransmitters, exerting an antihistaminic effect, and creating improvement of various symptoms. Other medications that are beneficial in the treatment of CFIDS do not cause improvement in depressive disorder. The symptoms of depression in PWCs disappear or decrease significantly when overall symptom improvement is accomplished. Dependence on alcohol and psychiatric medications is commonly characteristic of depressives; it is unusual for PWCs to be able to tolerate alcohol or such medications.

6. Sleep disorders. Sleep disorder is a prominent symptom of both depression and CFIDS but the disorders are different in the two illnesses. Characteristic in CFIDS is the delayed onset of dreaming sleep, the opposite of findings in depression, which show abbreviated onset of dreaming, and alpha-EEG sleep anomaly, which is also not known to be present in depression. Additional findings in CFIDS but not in depression include breathing difficulties, involuntary leg movements, increase in certain interleukin levels, and a drop in natural killer cell activity during sleep.

7. Psychological and neuropsychological testing. The Minnesota Multiphasic Personality Inventory (MMPI), widely used to diagnose psychological/psychiatric disorders, shows different findings for MDD and CFIDS. Linda Miller Iger, Ph.D., of the Chronic Fatigue Syndrome Institute in Anaheim Hills,

California, has found a unique MMPI profile for PWCs consisting of elevation of scales 1, 2, 3, 4, 7, and 8. Although it is beyond the scope of this chapter to describe this profile in detail, the significance of this finding is that it has not been seen in any other type of disorder, including depression, malingering, hypochondriasis, or other chronic illnesses. Thus, the MMPI is a useful tool for differentiating between CFIDS and depression. Scores on certain subtests of the Wechsler Adult Intelligence Scale-Revised are markedly decreased, and the IQ scores of PWCs are generally markedly decreased as compared to pre-morbid IQ scores. Performance of PWCs on certain neuropsychological tests is significantly impaired. These findings help us to distinguish between CFIDS and depressive disorders. Additionally, depressives tend to underestimate their performance on tests, probably due to decreased self-esteem and feelings of worthlessness. By contrast PWCs overestimate their abilities, most likely basing their expectations on their pre-morbid abilities and levels of functioning.

8. Contagion. Although it is unknown how CFIDS is spread, there have been cluster outbreaks of the syndrome for many years and the disease may be contagious, especially in its early stages. Depression is not known to be contagious or to occur in clusters.

9. Exercise intolerance. Exercise intolerance is characteristic of CFIDS but not of MDD. PWCs who exercise will generally experience a return or intensification of symptoms. Although those with MDD may be reluctant to exercise, their symptoms are generally improved by an exercise program.

10. Course of the illness. CFIDS tends to persist for many years even when treated, which is not generally characteristic of MDD. CFIDS tends to follow a waxing and waning pattern not usually seen with depression.

11. History. Most PWCs do not report a history of mood disorder in themselves or in their families, whereas the opposite is often true in MDD.

12. Other differences between MDD and CFIDS are related to age at onset and other demographic characteristics. Depression occurs increasingly with age; the age range for CFIDS is childhood to late adulthood with a predominance of cases in the middle years (thirties and forties). Those in certain professions are believed to be at greater risk of developing CFIDS, a phenomenon not found in MDD.

To summarize, chronic fatigue in and of itself is a common complaint and may be symptomatic of any number of problems; chronic fatigue *syndrome* is a distinct illness of which fatigue is one of myriad symptoms. Depression is a symptom of CFIDS but not its cause. Immune abnormalities and other findings and characteristics of CFIDS are not known to be found in mood disorders such as depression. Most PWCs were emotionally stable and not depressed prior to the onset of CFIDS. Those in the medical professions and the media who have confused the two disorders would do well to revise their thinking based on the preponderance of evidence that the two disorders are distinct. As one PWC commented, "This is not depression. I was never depressed until I got CFS. I was in love with life before I got sick."

(Note: This summary of the differences between CFIDS and MDD are based upon my clinical observations and on the work of such researchers and clinicians as Drs. Bastien, Goldstein, Hickie, Iger, Jacobson, Mena, Moldofsky, Sandman, and Wakefield.)

FINALLY, A LABEL

It is well-established that the mere fact of *knowing what hurts you has an inherent curative value.*
Hans Selye, M.D., *The Stress of Life*

Obtaining a diagnosis is a good news-bad news proposition. The good news: this is a physical, organic illness. "I'm not crazy. There's a name for this miserable condition. I have something other people have as well. This compact label replaces the long, difficult description of what's wrong. I was right to listen to my body; it really is telling me something is wrong. I have some control now that I know what I'm dealing with." One patient said, "I was so relieved to know I *had* something." A diagnosis gives us permission to be sick and offers validation of our complaints. It helps to explain the peculiar symptoms and sensations and alters our perspective on our lives and life changes. I summarized the initial postdiagnostic double bind in my journal: "Oh good, I'm really sick. Oh shit, I'm really sick."

The "honeymoon period," the initial relief of having obtained a diagnosis, is short-lived, and we are left once again to deal with the symptoms, the disruption, the lack of understanding of those around us. And we wonder, "Knowing is good—but now what do I do to become well again?" realizing that the answer to that question is not included in the diagnosis. We are labeled, put into a cubbyhole: I am a PWC, a Person with Chronic Fatigue Immune Dysfunction Syndrome. And the aftershock: the illness is real. It isn't going to go away overnight, if at all. I will have to make many changes in order to cope and maximize recovery potential; these changes will involve considerable sacrifice. Having obtained a diagnosis becomes a mixed blessing—first relief and then acknowledgment of the forthcoming journey into a different unknown.

Acknowledging CFIDS means losing a large degree of control over one's life. The illness continues to be unpredictable and unwelcome. The diagnosis brings with it a sense of betrayal, anger at one's body, feelings of fear and insecurity. And the inevitable question: *Why me?* The emotional aspects of diagnosis are varied and confusing as we ride the emotional roller coaster: denial, shock, truth, disbelief, numbness, anger, relief. We don't go through these emotions in any particular order and keep returning to the ones that are most difficult. Since the illness is chronic, its emotional effects continue and change with time.

COMMUNICATING THE DIAGNOSIS TO THE PATIENT

The way the diagnosis is communicated by the doctor can have a profound influence on the patient. Norman Cousins asked,

"Is it possible to communicate negative information in such a way that it is received by the patient as a challenge rather than as a death sentence?" Many physicians tell CFIDS patients such things as, "Just accept this and go on with your life," or "You have a chronic illness. There's nothing I can do for you. It will probably never go away." This is incomplete information, delivered with a closed-minded attitude.

CFIDS is not a death sentence but it may be a life sentence. Once a diagnosis has been made, it is far more constructive to discuss options, various treatment modalities and coping mechanisms, and the hope for a cure in the future. Physicians should try to motivate their patients, working together toward symptom alleviation. A dose of hope delivered along with the diagnosis is vital. Newly diagnosed PWCs need to hear such statements as, "You have quite a struggle ahead of you, but there is hope. We can experiment with treatments to see what works for you. You will probably get better over time and you may or may not fully recover. Numerous resources are available to you."

Despite the lack of a cure or even a reliable treatment program, patients should consult only competent, open-minded physicians and continue to stay well-informed about CFIDS theories and treatment possibilities. Patients who remain actively involved in treatment are more likely to do well than those who crawl back under the covers.

Chapter 5

✦

Symptoms

THE SYMPTOMS OF CFIDS vary among patients, and in individual patients over time. As new symptoms crop up, we may find it hard to determine whether they are part of the syndrome or something unrelated. The illness often begins with an odd assortment of symptoms, later joined or replaced by others. Early in the illness the PWC is likely to experience swollen lymph glands, frequent infections and illnesses, fever and chills, sore throat, depression, and persistent headaches and myalgias. As time goes on, additional symptoms such as neurological symptoms and nausea may develop or become worse. The pattern varies widely among individuals.

Betty, a PWC, reported:

> I had laryngitis all the month of December. I had to make long-distance calls at work, and I could hardly talk. Later in December I noticed difficulty in walking. My legs felt heavy and they ached. I thought, "This is weird. I feel like I've been running around a tennis court for two or three hours, when in reality I've been sitting at my desk." My legs ached, I took labored steps and thought, "I'm not old enough for this to be happening." I didn't know what it was but I ignored it because there were things I had to take care of. My throat hurt all the time, I ached; I was still pushing myself.

51

In my case, the illness began with a bout of what I thought was the flu or a "bug": fatigue, malaise, and lethargy. Within a few months these symptoms were joined by others: tinnitus (ringing in the ears), sore throat, equilibrium problems, irritability, morning nausea, weight gain, and shortness of breath. Additional symptoms developed over time: lymph node tenderness, unusual headaches, a tendency to become "overloaded" easily by activity or any type of sensory stimulation, brief periods of severe depression, a periodic inability to find the right words as I spoke, and slowed speech and thinking. I tried to ignore other odd symptoms: photosensitivity, transient facial numbness, night sweats, "broken thermostat" (random sensitivity to heat and/or cold), heart palpitations, and general weakness. I popped vitamins and continued the hectic pace of my life as mother, therapist, workshop presenter, college instructor, and, jogger. I attempted to ignore or overcome my symptoms because they didn't make any sense and because they got in my way. I did what I had always done: I pushed hard and fought aggressively.

In retrospect my approach didn't make much sense. Dogs have the good sense to rest an injured paw by using only the other three until healing occurs. I used to think symptoms were a signal to do *more* of what I was already doing. As is common in early CFIDS, I didn't talk to many people about what was happening to me because I felt too wimpy, vulnerable, and crazy to risk others judging the situation. I simply wasn't allowed to have such things happen to me. I'm not a weakling, hypochondriac, somatizer, hysteric, or victim to whom such things happen. In fact, as a psychotherapist, I'm a provider of help—not a recipient! So I tried to ignore my symptoms, hoping they'd disappear. Sometimes they did, only to return accompanied by other symptoms.

Other PWCs relate similar stories in which various unusual, bewildering symptoms occur, disappear, and reappear. In the past many had experienced allergies, colds, and viral illnesses from which they had typically recovered within a few weeks. They assumed that their new symptoms would follow a similar course. But all of us have been astounded at the variety, unpredictability, and duration of the symptoms we have experienced. Toni Jeffreys described the symptoms as a "cafeteria in a nightmare" with each patient experiencing a "horrendous array of horrors" (1982).

The following list of symptoms is grouped into three general categories with approximate percentages of PWCs who experience them. These percentages are based upon information reported by Drs. Bell, Fudenberg, Goldstein, Jessop, Komaroff, Peterson, and two surveys (Kansas City and Phoenix). An asterisk indicates that no statistics are currently available. Overlapping categories are used for the sake of convenience: in some cases it is difficult to assign a symptom to a particular category when its cause is unclear (e.g., headache or muscle weakness). Many of the symptoms listed in the general/physical and emotional/psychological categories may actually be caused by neurological dysfunction.

General or Physical Symptoms

fatigue, often accompanied by nonrestorative sleep, generally worsened by exertion: 95–100%
nausea: 60–90%
irritable bowel syndrome (diarrhea, nausea, gas, abdominal pain): 60–90%
chronic sore throat: 50–90%
fevers/chills/sweats: 50–90%
muscle and/or joint pain, neck pain: 50–90%
bladder/prostate problems, frequent urination: 20–95%
low blood pressure: 86%
recurrent illness (flu-like illness, various infections): 70–85%
malaise: 80%
heat/cold intolerance: 75–80%
painful and/or swollen lymph nodes: 50–80%
systemic yeast/fungal infection: 30–80%
fungal infection of skin and nails: 71%
weight gain: 50–70%
increased/severe PMS (premenstrual syndrome): 70%

low-grade fevers/feeling hot often: 55–70%
swelling, fluid retention: 55–70%
shortness of breath: 30–70%
subnormal body temperature: 65%
severe allergies: 40–65%
sensitivities to medicines, inhalants, odors, and
    foods: 25–65%
difficulty swallowing: 55–60%
heart palpitations: 40–60%
sinus pain: 56%
rash or flushing of face: 35–45%
chest pain: 40%
hair loss: 20–35%
eye pain: 30%
pressure at the base of the skull: 30%
weight loss: 20–30%
tendency to bruise easily: 25%
vomiting: 20%
endometriosis*
dryness of mouth, eyes*
pressure sensation behind eyes*
frequent canker sores*
cough*
Temporomandibular Joint (TMJ) syndrome (jaw pain
    or locking)*
mitral valve prolapse*
carpal tunnel syndrome*
serious cardiac rhythm disturbances*
pyriform muscle syndrome, causing sciatica*
impotence*
thyroid inflammation*
periodontal (gum) disease*
hypoglycemia or hypoglycemia-like symptoms*
swelling of nasal passages*
first trimester miscarriage*

Neurological/Central Nervous System-Related Symptoms

confusion; inability to think clearly: 75–100%

concentration/attention deficit: 70–100%

sleep disorder/disturbance (insomnia, unrestorative sleep, unusual nightmares): 65–100%

muscle weakness: 85–95%

headache: 75–95% (daily headache: 50%)

memory problems (especially short-term memory): 80–90%

photosensitivity: 65–90%

dysequilibrium, spatial disorientation, dizziness, vertigo: 60–90%

spaceyness, light-headedness: 75–85%

muscle twitching, involuntary movements: 55–80%

aphasia (inability to find the right word, saying the wrong word) and/or dyscalculia (difficulty with numbers): 75–80%

alcohol intolerance: 45–75%

seizure-like episodes: 70% (seizures: 2%)

coordination problems/clumsiness: 60%

paresthesias (numbness, tingling or other odd sensations in face and/or extremeties): 25–60%

visual disturbance (scratchiness, blurring of vision, "floaters"—harmless spots behind the lens of the eye): 45–55%

episodic hyperventilation: 40–45%

fainting or blackouts: 40%

strange taste in mouth (bitter, metallic): 25%

temporary paralysis after sleeping: 20%

earache: 20%

decreased libido*

hallucinations*

alteration of taste, smell, hearing*

tinnitus (ringing in the ears)*

Emotional/Psychological Symptoms

anxiety 70–90%
mood swings, excessive irritability, overreaction: 70–90%
depression: 65–90%
personality change: 55–75%
panic attacks: 30–40%
isolative tendencies*

*Indicates no statistics available at this time.

These figures represent a range of percentages of reported symptoms in different studies. Patients do not necessarily experience these symptoms all the time. In most cases only one-third to one-half of those reporting individual symptoms indicated that they experienced the symptom at all times. In my survey of the Phoenix area group, figures were compiled to indicate the average total number of symptoms each patient experienced all of the time (11 symptoms) and the average total number of symptoms experienced by each patient some of the time (18.6 symptoms).

PWCs may experience symptoms other than those listed above. Some of the symptoms reported may have been experienced prior to the onset of CFIDS in a milder or different form. Additionally, other illnesses or conditions may exist simultaneously with CFIDS, complicating the diagnostic problems and often causing lack of clarity as to which symptoms are attributable to which conditions. The major symptoms in each group are discussed below in some detail.

GENERAL OR PHYSICAL SYMPTOMS

Fatigue

A hallmark of CFIDS, and often the first symptom to appear, is chronic fatigue. To the healthy, fatigue means tiredness, feeling worn out, or needing a nap. CFIDS-related fatigue is of a different magnitude: a phenomenon that spans feeling debilitated, disabled, exhausted, drained, washed out, weak, wasted, zapped, and unable to function mentally or physically. The degree of fatigue varies over time. CFIDS fatigue defies description and cannot be measured.

CFIDS fatigue is often accompanied by a sense of feeling totally unable to cope, along with general malaise, or feeling "sick all over." In some cases the fatigue waxes and wanes, often unpredictably; in others, severe fatigue is constant. Some patients are literally unable to get out of bed. Some describe the experience of waking up, showering and dressing, and then getting back into bed, having drained the day's energy supply in these simple activities. What used to be preparation for the day can become the day's only activities; even the simple act of brushing one's teeth can become a monumental chore. Although this may sound dramatic and exaggerated to a healthy individual, it is all too real and very discouraging to the PWC.

Fatigue may be worsened by exercise and by physical or emotional exertion. Although some PWCs find that stretching exercises or yoga are helpful in alleviating fatigue, others are unable to exert themselves even minimally without danger of collapse. Exercise tolerance varies considerably among PWCs.

Just as the Eskimos have many different words for "snow," we need more precise words for the phenomenon we call "fatigue" to indicate the type of fatigue and its severity. At times I feel extremely fatigued but not sleepy in a way that is difficult to explain to others. One PWC in her seventies said that at certain times of the day she would "just need to go flat." She didn't need to sleep but only to rest in a horizontal position for about thirty minutes before resuming even mild activity.

Many PWCs describe a type of fatigue referred to as "sensory overload," which is described more completely in the "Cognitive/Central Nervous System Symptoms" discussion. Sensory input of a specific type or of a combination of types (noise, light, motion, etc.) becomes overwhelming and debilitating.

Sleep does not necessarily relieve CFIDS-related fatigue. Although the perceived need for sleep may be great, even many hours of sleep may not be refreshing, and the PWC may awaken still tired. In his book *Waiting to Live*, Gregg Fisher described his need for sleep:

I have often slept for twelve hours or more, only to wake up feeling much sicker than I did the night before. I believe part of the reason for this is that I did not get a good night's sleep. Sometimes I wake up two or three times during the middle of the night, totally disoriented. Other nights I toss and turn so much, I use more energy than I gain. (1987, p. 44)

Extreme fatigue may be accompanied by an inability to sleep. The problems include difficulty falling asleep, early awakening, or frequent awakenings during the night. One patient complained that she felt tired all the time but was unable to sleep more than a few hours per night. Inactivity compounds the problem, but increased activity may lead to relapse.

Living with constant or cycling fatigue is at best difficult and at worst devastating to one's lifestyle. Kyle reports:

I pretty much came to a full halt. I had lived a full life, I was going twelve hours a day. Now that I'm sick, I work four hours a day and am pooped when I get home. I'm in my recliner all evening. If I push myself I can go out maybe one or two nights a week, but I pay for it dearly. The next day, I'm done, that's it; I'm sicker. It's a real effort for me to do anything. I'm too tired and lazy to eat well; I'd rather stay in my chair.

I am tempted to open a treatment center called "Nappers Anonymous." There are books about all sorts of addictions— negative ones, such as chemical dependency, smoking, compulsive sex, gambling—and positive ones, such as jogging, aerobics, and health foods. The books about the former tell you how to get rid of the habits, and about the latter, how to develop them: what to wear, how to do it, and how often. My most recent addiction is sleeping, but I can't find much material about it. I do, however, have several suitable sleeping outfits complemented by nonmatching socks. I don't have trouble figuring out when to sleep, but sometimes the "how" eludes me. A "sleeper's handbook" would be helpful, perhaps *The Joy of Napping* or *The Art of Sleeping*.

Aches and pains

> I'm old too soon, yet young too long;
> Could Swift himself have planned it droller?
> *Timor vitae conturbat me;*
> Another day, another dolor.
>   *Ogden Nash,* "A Man Can Complain, Can't He?"

Lots of things hurt. Ellen describes waking up each morning wondering, "What's going to hurt today?" Sometimes it was her arms, other times her legs, and sometimes she hurt all over. On rare days, nothing hurt. Her problem had been diagnosed as arthritis, but her other puzzling symptoms didn't fit with that label, and CFIDS was ultimately diagnosed.

Betty says:

> I'd pushed [the pain] aside because it was something I didn't want to come to grips with, something I told myself wasn't happening. All of a sudden I had acquired arthritic symptoms. I started swelling. My hands, my legs, my joints, between the rib cage and the sternum. They took thermograms. It's been one test after another. I don't know if it's arthritis or symptoms of arthritis attributable to [CFIDS]. My doctor doesn't know. If I don't take my arthritis drug, I feel worse; I ache all over. Every now and then I test myself by going a couple of days without it, and I start hurting. I know enough now to know it's not psychosomatic. It hurts; I ache all over.

PWCs describe various types of pain: in their joints, muscles, lymph nodes (notably those in the neck and armpits), and throat. In some cases pain is the predominant symptom, and the illness may be diagnosed as fibromyalgia or fibrositis. Some PWCs report increased pain when they are most fatigued. The onset of even mild pain can serve as a warning sign: time to stop and rest.

Many PWCs complain of localized sore spots, often called tender points or trigger points. Even gentle pressure on one of these spots can cause anything from a wince to a trip right through the ceiling.

Patients may complain of swollen or tender lymph nodes. There may be extreme soreness without any swelling, or slight swelling noticeable to the patient but unremarkable to the physician. Soreness in the nodes in the back of the neck is commonly reported; some patients describe difficulty turning their necks. Such neck pain may be accompanied by headache, sinus pain, or eye pain.

The headaches described by CFIDS patients are of varying types, falling into either the "general/physical" or "central nervous system" symptom categories. Some are migraine-like, in that the headache is unilateral (on only one side of the head, as migraines often are), and sometimes accompanied by nausea and sensitivity to light and noise. Others describe headaches accompanied by severe pain behind the eyes and/or sinus pain. Patients may refer to their headaches as "CFIDS headaches" to distinguish them from "normal" (previously experienced) headaches. CFIDS headaches may last for several hours or several days. They may develop in one side of the head, moving to the other side on the following day. Here, too, the patterns vary considerably as does the pain level. Excruciating ones have been described as Lizzie Borden headaches, chisels-behind-the-eyes headaches, and "ten pounds of shit in a five pound bag" headaches, the latter referring to the sensation of increased pressure.

Sore throat is another common complaint: the pain ranges from mild to severe among patients and in some individuals over time. Like other aches, a mild sore throat may serve as a warning signal heralding a "crash." Severe exacerbations of CFIDS may be accompanied by a strep-like sore throat.

Some patients without sore throat complain of difficulty swallowing, probably caused by swelling in the lymph nodes. Those with this complaint may have to cut their food into small bites and crush large pills and vitamins. Some patients complain of choking or a fear of choking.

Allergies

About two-thirds of the PWCs I surveyed indicated a history of allergies. Most of them, as well as many previously nonallergic patients, report more severe allergic symptoms and an increased sensitivity to various environmental substances, foods, and plants. It has been speculated that all CFIDS patients have allergies and sensitivities of which some are not aware. Many PWCs are sensitive to the odors of perfumes, exhaust fumes, cleaning products, and other chemicals. Exposure to these substances may produce overall discomfort, nasal congestion, headache, equilibrium problems, and a return or increase of other symptoms.

Some PWCs report new sensitivities to food additives, such as preservatives, colorings, and flavorings. Some report particular sensitivity to sulfites (commonly found in diet soda, wine, prepared foods, produce, and fresh or frozen fish). A few patients report a negative response to sodium benzoate or to aspartame (Nutrasweet).

Sensitivity to temperature extremes

Many PWCs become extremely sensitive to heat and/or cold. Kyle says, "I get cold. Other people say they're hot, and I say I'm freezing. I feel like an idiot carrying a sweater around all the time. My bones are cold."

It's like having a broken thermostat. Some patients can tolerate only a very limited temperature range, becoming unusually uncomfortable with small variations in either direction. Like Kyle, they may feel cold most of the time, even when others feel warm or (less commonly) just the reverse. This problem may be attributable to effects of the illness on a particular part of the brain, causing metabolic and other problems.

Low body temperature, fever and sweats

Subnormal body temperature is reported by many patients. In some cases the problem is thyroid-related, although routine thyroid tests may yield normal results. Some doctors routinely prescribe thyroid medication for patients with low body temperatures and other symptoms of hypothyroidism, even when test results are within the normal range, while others disapprove of this practice.

A possible explanation for low body temperature was offered by John Reed, M.D., who stated at a Phoenix support group meeting in March 1988: "Microorganisms do things to slow the body down to make a happy home for themselves." Viruses are quite fond of and replicate best at temperatures slightly below normal body temperature.

My body temperature jumps around madly at times. One day I remarked to a friend that my temperature had jumped from 96.6° to 99.4° in just a few hours. (His advice: "When it gets to 100, SELL!") Someone whose body temperature is "subnormal" (below 98°) will feel feverish at a "normal" temperature of 98.6°.

Some PWCs report low-grade fevers either intermittently or constantly over long periods of time. They may experience night sweats resembling hot flashes: an abrupt rush of heat and sweating, especially in the upper portion of the body.

Weight gain and loss

When CFIDS was thought to be chronic Epstein-Barr Virus syndrome, the assumption was that most patients would lose weight, as is the tendency with EBV-caused mononucleosis. Weight gain has turned out to be a more common problem in CFIDS. What a rip-off! Chronic illness is enough of a problem without causing weight gain. It seems that those of us who have fought the battle of the bulge all our lives have gained weight during the time we have had CFIDS, and the "skinnies" tend to lose weight. How has this virus (or causative agent, or whatever) found our weakest, most vulnerable spots and learned to sabotage them?

In our society, being overweight is equated with a weak-willed, out-of-control person who has "let herself go" (go where? to the refrigerator?). Stigma city: the assumption is that being overweight signals emotional weakness rather than a physiological problem. It is common for PWCs to experience weight gains of 30–60 pounds during CFIDS, and some patients have gained in the vicinity of 100 pounds. Although the weight gain is attributable in part to inactivity or to increased carbohydrate consumption due to certain cravings, many PWCs experience weight gain without increased food consumption or any significant change in eating habits. Weight change is another baffling CFIDS symptom, one most likely attributable to altered metabolism or alterations in brain chemistry and functioning.

Many PWCs experience decreased self-esteem, helplessness, and anger regarding weight gain. "I have no control over my weight," remarked one. "It's on its own little program." Another lamented, "I'm heavier than I've ever been in my life. I've gained a great deal of weight and am so dissatisfied with my size, but my doctor told me not to worry about it. The weight will come off later, he says." This gaining trend is a leading cause of High School Reunion Syndrome (HSRS), which is summarized as "I don't want them to see me like this."

In an article called, "Weight-ing to Lose," (her title a likely takeoff on Gregg Fisher's *Waiting to Live*), Connie Steitz Fox laments her increasing girth with mirth. She claimed that "even a dead person's metabolism is higher than mine" (*The CFIDS Chronicle*, August 1988). I have speculated bitterly that any illness that causes years of daily morning nausea coupled with weight gain is likely to result in the birth of a large mammal.

Some PWCs have lost weight, generally those who have been involuntarily underweight all their lives. In extreme cases, individuals have become almost skeletal in appearance. This excessive weight loss, although problematic for them, is unlikely to elicit understanding and sympathy in our society, which values thinness.

Bladder and urinary problems

Interstitial cystitis is an inflammation of the space between the bladder lining and muscle. Men as well as women may develop this condition, which causes pain on urination and sometimes during sexual intercourse. Unlike a bladder or urinary tract infection, interstitial cystitis is not caused by bacteria, so antibiotics are not helpful in treatment. Larrian Gillespie, M.D., (1986) believes that such cofactors as hormones, certain drugs, and viruses may play causal roles; additional cofactors, if any, remain unknown. It may be an autoimmune disease. Gillespie regards interstitial cystitis as an environmental disease that is progressive, in which the bladder has become ulcerated and scarred. It is treatable but not curable. Chemical sensitivity may contribute to this problem. Prostatitis, an inflammation and/or swelling of the prostate gland, has been reported by some male CFIDS patients and is treatable.

Abdominal pain and digestive problems

Jenny reports having been diagnosed by various specialists as having not only irritable bowel syndrome but also arthritis, Ménière's disease, anxiety disorder, and depression before anyone put the symptoms together and saw CFIDS (like the story of the blind men and the elephant). This situation is not unique.

Irritable bowel syndrome has been diagnosed in many PWCs with such symptoms as nausea, gassiness and bloating, diarrhea, abdominal cramps, and constipation. Like other symptoms, these may be constant or intermittent.

Yeast overgrowth

Candida albicans, or yeast, is normally present in the body, particularly in the intestinal tract. Under certain conditions, yeast cells proliferate out of control in the intestines and elsewhere in the body, causing a host of uncomfortable symptoms including rectal or vaginal itching, gas and bloating, feelings of spaceyness or disorientation, and other symptoms often associated with CFIDS. Although the relationship between CFIDS and yeast overgrowth is not clear, some practitioners believe that the two often occur simultaneously. Others view candidiasis as a "fad" diagnosis, as hypoglycemia once was, for example.

This diagnosis remains controversial and unproven. However, many CFIDS patients report feeling better on an antiyeast diet, one that eliminates sugars, alcohol, other refined carbohydrates, and sometimes yeast and dairy products.

Other illnesses

Some CFIDS patients report that they have developed a series of infections and illnesses, especially early in the illness, and are prone to catch "whatever is going around." One woman complained, "I came down with two different kinds of flu in one month. I threw up; I had diarrhea. I passed out." Another said, "I get everything that comes down the pike." Others state that they have been less prone to catching other illnesses. It is common for other illnesses and infections to appear in early CFIDS but to become less frequent over time.

CFIDS and pregnancy

In many cases pregnancy brings about a remission of CFIDS symptoms, starting several weeks after conception and lasting until several weeks after delivery. In some cases a permanent remission seems to take place. Anecdotal reports indicate a possibly higher-than-average rate of miscarriage. Babies born to PWCs generally thrive and do well. The child may be at increased risk of birth defects, even fatal ones, or of developing CFIDS if the mother contracted this illness during her pregnancy, especially in the first trimester. However, there have been no formal studies of CFIDS and pregnancy, so this information is speculative and is based upon the observations of physicians who treat PWCs, including Drs. Behan, Cheney, Hyde, and Jones.

NEUROLOGICAL SYMPTOMS

Initially viewed as a viral disorder and later as immune system dysfunction, CFIDS is now being considered a neurological illness, or a psychoneuroimmunological one. (Rather than be intimidated by that word, take it apart. Its components are psychological, neurological, and immunological—a description of the interactions of all the parts of the body affected by CFIDS.) Neurological testing and patient reports reveal numerous neurological/cognitive deficits, reflected in lower-than-expected scores on tests of intelligence, performance, achievement, and neurological functioning.

PWCs describe neurological/cognitive functions in interesting terms:

I've got cotton in my synapses

Something is chewing on my wiring

I'm reacting backwards to everything

I feel like someone spilled Coke in my keyboard

I've got brain fog

This feels like Alzheimer's, or maybe just "Halfheimer's"

My brain is on strike

I become so disoriented. Sometimes I don't know where I am, even when I'm in my own neighborhood

I feel like a camera lens that can't focus

I feel like a VCR on "pause"

I've been short-circuited

I feel like there's an infection in my brain. It just isn't working right

Neurological problems include visual disturbances, vestibular (balance) problems, numbness and tingling feelings, light-headedness, abnormal movements, seizures or seizure-like episodes, difficulty concentrating, impaired short-term memory, and other cognitive impairments to be discussed in the next section. Such symptoms may appear with the onset of CFIDS but often emerge weeks or months later. Neurological deficits are acute in many patients, waxing and waning in severity over time, and absent or mild in others. Sheila Bastien, M.D., refers to CFIDS as an "atypical organic brain syndrome" (April 1990).

Many doctors dismiss such complaints as manifestations of emotional problems or hypochondriasis. However, the consistency among patient reports of such symptoms and the lack of evidence of previous psychiatric problems among CFIDS patients suggest that these neurological symptoms are CFIDS-related.

Stephen Straus, M.D., of the National Institute of Health acknowledged these abnormalities but found them to be of uncertain importance (March 1988). Straus has tended to downplay the significance of this syndrome and seems to under-estimate the seriousness of reported neurological problems and clinical findings.

Although caution should be applied in drawing conclusions from the current findings, patient reports and test results are sufficiently abnormal to generate further research.

Cognitive problems

> Unusual cognitive complaints are, increasingly to
> me, the single most important symptom.
>   Paul Cheney, M.D.
>   (*The CFIDS Chronicle*, November 1990, p. 8)

Each of us has developed a concept of how we normally func-tion based on past abilities and characteristics. When our brains aren't working right or functioning as they used to, we become frustrated and frightened and fear loss of identity. Cog-nitive problems include difficulty with speech (e.g., with word-finding ability, word transposition or using the wrong word—often an incorrect term from the right category, such as saying "hot" when we meant to say "cold"), unusual headaches, diffi-culty with numbers and mathematical computations, problem-solving difficulty, attention deficit, problems absorbing and encoding information, directional problems, gross and fine motor problems, abstract reasoning deficits, sequencing problems, and difficulty gauging distances and time (visual/spatial problems).

Betty describes her neurological deficits and related fears:

> I would have to read and reread because I had forgotten what I had read. For a person who's doing research and writing for professional journals and the media, this became disconcert-ing, and I was scared. I was so frightened that I did not want to tell my family, my coworkers, anybody. I thought this must be presenile dementia; I had the telltale signs. At meetings, I was quiet, because it was so difficult for me to concentrate; I didn't know how to say what I wanted to say. I couldn't always

figure out which words to use. I became reclusive because I was afraid others would find out.

When I was driving, I'd have to force myself to focus so I wouldn't wreck me and my new car. I'd forget where I was, where I was supposed to be going, and why. I was afraid to pull over because someone might find me and discover what had happened. It was hard for me to remember where my office was. When I remembered and got there, I wondered what I was supposed to be doing and I was afraid to ask my secretary. My aide asked, "Are you all right?" I thought, "Dear God, this is it. I can't continue." I didn't know if I was going to break down or what.

Many patients report similar experiences of being unable to ascertain their whereabouts in familiar territory, rereading because of an inability to absorb, losing track of a train of thought, or forgetting how to perform simple tasks.

Susan reported a fairly typical experience in which she became lost while driving in her own neighborhood and asked her five-year-old son to direct her home, pretending it was a game. Another patient whose impairment was more consistent gave up driving and now relies on others for transportation. She no longer trusted herself behind the wheel of a car because of poor judgment and a tendency to become lost in familiar areas. Those who experience this strange phenomenon feel embarrassed and dumb and are often reluctant to tell others, even their doctors. One patient explained, "I feel drunk when I drive," and another stated, "I feel like I'm in another dimension. It takes all my concentration to drive."

We live in a society where faster is better, and slow performance is not okay. PWCs react more slowly and speak more slowly, like 45-rpm records being played at 33⅓. We fear that others will notice, that we will be ridiculed, lose our jobs and lose our identities as intelligent, functional human beings. One woman said sadly, "My life is not the same. I have an above-average thinking process and now I feel so dull and slow. My mind is no longer sharp."

"My brain is broken," laments Kyle. "I can't even say things that are important to me any more. That's when I get angry. I'd answer the phone at work and then couldn't remember who was calling; I'd have to ask someone two or three times and still not remember."

"I depended on this wonderful tool that I have, my brain, and it just doesn't work very well any more," reports a now-unemployed patient who has neither the energy nor the cognitive ability to work any longer.

"My memory doesn't work well, my brain doesn't work well, and I get spacey and lose pieces of information," says one PWC, and Betty adds:

> The forgetting is hard. I lose track of myself. I test myself periodically to see if my mind is still working. When I can't recall something, I feel devastated. I used to have an excellent memory; it was frightening when it failed me. I was losing myself. All of a sudden, I didn't know who I was, or what I was becoming. I tried to train my mind to remember; I made lists every day. I was hopelessly lost; I couldn't think. I couldn't read or write or knit because I kept losing track. All of a sudden my mind was gone. It was awful.

Reading had been an important leisure pastime for Betty, who experienced a double loss: inability to work, and inability to pursue an enjoyable pastime. (Update: one year later, Betty reports considerable improvement, although she has not yet returned to work.)

Normally an avid reader, I use my comprehension level as a cognitive-function barometer. When I was sickest I had no desire to read. With a slight improvement in health, I was able to read fiction or humor but often lost track or didn't get the jokes. I joked feebly that since our recall and earning abilities are impaired, we PWCs are able to read the same book over and over; at best, it's vaguely familiar the second time around. (Obviously, my impaired sense of humor is another barometer.) As my health and cognitive functioning improved over time, I regained my comprehension level and became able to resume my former reading habits. My cognitive improvement has been fairly consistent over time but is still mildly affected by exacerbations.

Several PWCs echo the statement seen on some bumper stickers and T-shirts: "Of all the things I've lost, I miss my mind the most." Knowing that adequate cognitive functioning will most likely return over time is helpful during relapses, when it seems our minds are gone forever.

In her well-known article in *Rolling Stone*, Hilary Johnson wrote about her inability to concentrate, hold a conversation in a group, use appropriate and often simple words, sustain a train of thought, and recall such familiar things as names of her friends and schools she had attended. She described such behavioral errors as picking up the wrong object (a comb instead of a pen), trying to replace a drawer in a space that was actually a shelf, and being unable to fasten her seatbelt on an airplane (July 1987). Another PWC described forgetting how to turn on the headlights of his car, and many report similar inabilities to do common, daily "simple stuff."

Many describe this confused state as brain-spin or trance-like states of altered perception. "I feel dizzy, light-headed; my brain spins. My vision changes a lot; sometimes things look closer than they really are or everything will look unusually crisp and clear," says one. "I get an intense buzzing feeling throughout my system. It varies in intensity. It's not a noise, it's a drugged-like feeling, it's systemic. It's in my head mostly, but I can feel it throughout. It affects my thought processes," says another.

Many report distorted thinking and unusual thought patterns and images they never experienced prior to the onset of CFIDS. They describe vivid, often disturbing dreams that may be accompanied by strong sensations lasting into their waking hours. Phillip Rubin, M.D., described "altered perception in waking and sleeping" (1988).

Photosensitivity

Most PWCs are sensitive to light. Many avoid bright sunlight, wear dark sunglasses outdoors, and keep indoor lighting dim. Additionally, many are sensitive to fluorescent lighting, describing it as harsh, eerie, and disturbing. Fluorescent lighting sensitivity may be associated with balance disorders.

Symptoms associated with exposure to bright light include dizziness and other equilibrium problems, nausea, sensory "overload," and headache. One patient reports feeling "blinded" by bright sunlight, needing to cling to a friend's arm for support. Although some patients are acutely aware of this problem, others recognize it or associate it with CFIDS only when asked if light sensitivity is experienced.

Vision problems

David J. Browning, M.D., a North Carolina ophthalmologist, states that numerous vision problems have been reported, ranging from mild to severe: floaters (harmless floating spots behind the lens of the eye), transient blurred vision, transient double vision, extreme light sensitivity, burning, and pain. A very small minority of patients may develop serious conditions such as multifocal choroiditis and panuveitis, which are inflammations thought to result from viral infections.

Although the patient may report experiencing the more common problems to an ophthalmologist, most of them are not readily apparent upon examination. Dr. Browning recommends seeking a doctor who takes such complaints seriously and is willing to initiate a trial-and-error approach to symptom treatment. He stresses that in most cases the eyes will appear normal upon examination, and that the problems may be due to "the immunoneurological problem causing the fatigue, inability to concentrate ('focus'), and increased sensitivity to noxious stimuli" (*The CFIDS Chronicle*, October 1988).

Vestibular (balance) problems

Included in this symptom category are: dizziness; vertigo; spatial disorientation; difficulty navigating (e.g., loss of balance, frequently bumping into things, or listing to one side); nausea, with or without vomiting; and tinnitus (ringing in the ears). These problems may be associated with feelings of anxiety, often accompanying phobias and panic disorders. Usually transient, these problems may fluctuate with other symptoms, but in a minority of patients, vestibular symptoms are constant.

"Medically, dizziness and vertigo are different," wrote Sara Reynolds, M.D., a Phoenix physician and PWC:

> *Dizziness* is the "spacey" feeling we sometimes get—possibly a feeling of falling or a feeling that things are going black, as if one were about to faint. On the other hand, *vertigo* is essentially a sensation of surrounding movement. The most severe vertigo leaves its victim holding onto the bed desperately, feeling that the bed is moving so violently that he will be pitched onto the floor.

She added that these sensations often occur with viral infection.

> Occasionally, *tinnitus* (ringing or buzzing in the ears) is associated with vertigo, and again the level of sound is usually not constant and varies from person to person, and from time to time. It may interfere with normal hearing and is usually unilateral (in one ear only).
>
> (*The CFS Bulletin*, May 1988)

Patients report a variety of sensations typical of vestibular disorders: a sense of unreality or disorientation, or of feeling "foggy" or "spacey," light-headedness, shortness of breath, episodic momentary loss of equilibrium, increased disorientation in the dark, inability to concentrate, increased distractibility, and a need to restrict motion to some degree. Some must remain perfectly still in bed; others are ambulatory but must restrict head movement, or may not do well on escalators, elevators, and some forms of transportation. These sensations are often described as trancelike and may be produced or worsened by certain types of motion, noise, odors, or bright light.

Harold Levinson, M.D., associates such sensations with malfunction of the cerebellar-vestibular system (CVS), which is responsible for processing and making sense of external sensory input to maintain orientation and balance. If this "filter" malfunctions, incoming messages become scrambled, resulting in the sensations described above. He discusses this concept at length in *Phobia Free* (1986) and spoke at the 1987 CFS Convention in Portland: "It's not just a balance problem. The inner ear system doesn't control just a balance and coordination output, but acts as a sort of a fine-tuner to the whole brain. It fine-tunes the whole sensory input, sort of like what a fine-tuner does to a TV set."

Levinson has tied certain learning disorders, many symptoms of anxiety, and many phobias to CVS dysfunction, reporting a corresponding decrease in self-esteem as these problems occur. Levinson believes that a viral illness such as mononucleosis can trigger vestibular problems, resulting in the symptoms reported by so many CFS patients: tripping, stumbling, dizziness, slurred speech, impaired coordination, and so on. He discussed blurry or scrambled input, which is not appropriately filtered or sorted out by the brain and results in distorted signals and thus confusion. Overload is the phenomenon of too much input, causing even small amounts of additional input to create exaggerated responses, resulting in an increase in vestibular symptoms.

Levinson described situations that are difficult for many CFIDS patients, such as shopping in crowded stores and being bombarded with motion, lights (which may be bright, fluorescent, and/or flickering), colors, shapes, odors (foods, perfumes, or cleaning solvents), people talking, music playing, and so on. This large amount of visual, auditory, and motion-related input results in overload and such symptoms as spaceyness, imbalance, disorientation, anxiety (sometimes with panic attacks), inability to navigate properly in space, stumbling or falling, hyperventilation, concentration impairment, nausea and vomiting, motion sickness, and mental fogginess. These symptoms, like most others, tend to wax and wane.

EMOTIONAL SYMPTOMS

The notion of mind-body duality or dichotomy has fallen into disfavor. Although we can distinguish some primarily physiologically-caused problems, such as a bone fracture, from emotional problems, such as depression following the loss of a loved one, emotional and physical problems are interrelated. So-called physical problems have psychological manifestations and vice versa. Illness is a function of the "mindbody," an integrated system.

When we seek medical help for symptoms whose "physical" cause cannot be found, we may be told that it is an "emotional" problem, that it is "all in our heads." What exactly does that mean? That we have fabricated symptoms? That we want them? That we are crazy? That we seek attention for imaginary ills? To so label an illness with both emotional and physical symptoms is inappropriate and insulting. Phrases such as "all in your head" and "mind over matter" add insult to illness. Emotional symptoms are no less real than physical ones.

Typical CFIDS-related emotions include depression, anxiety, anger, frustration, and disappointment. A majority of patients report mood swings that may be abrupt and are triggered by minor events or occur without apparent cause. These mood swings lead to out-of-control feelings; the way we react makes no sense to us. The reaction is out of proportion to the stimulus and is not typical of past responses.

We may call such mood swings "emotional overreaction," or being "too sensitive," or "going crazy over nothing." The overload phenomenon described earlier may help to explain such reactions. When an individual's tolerance threshold is low, any stimulus may become too much to process logically. Even healthy people experience busy, frustrating days during which minor incidents become major problems. This phenomenon in CFIDS, though, is radically different in kind and in degree. Our short fuses may result in sudden, intense angry outbursts, often surprising to others and to us. Angry outbursts may be triggered by the direct effect of a virus on the limbic system, a part of the brain thought to control anger and aggressive behavior. The situationally-induced helplessness and frustration of being ill may also trigger outbursts, which may be inappropriately directed at someone in the immediate environment, such as a spouse, family member, or co-worker. Exhaustion makes anger more difficult to direct constructively.

When PWCs are sickest, even the mildest frustration or sensory input is intolerable. Music or conversation (especially in combination) becomes grating. At such times we are more prone to react very strongly to any sort of demand, frustration, or problem. Our tolerance threshold is lowered considerably, and our responses to such events are often quite extreme—irrational, and often angry. The reactions we feel are out of proportion to the events.

The emotional aspects of CFIDS can be devastating and crazy-making because our reactions are not typical of us and don't make sense. Others in our environment may be more puzzled and disturbed by our emotional changes than by our other symptoms.

Anxiety

"I always feel nervous now, all the time," says Bill. "I'm nervous when I get up in the morning. I'm nervous right now. My nerves are so whacked out; maybe there's something actively attacking them."

"In response to almost nothing . . . my heart was pounding, my skin was burning, my anxiety level was skyrocketing," remarks Yolanda. "What the hell is the matter? I just can't handle stress. This is really guilt-provoking."

Other patients comment:

> My heart starts to pound, and I feel as if I'm going to pass out—for no reason! I can't figure out what causes this; I really don't feel anxious about anything in particular.

> I've never had this problem before. Sure, I've gotten uptight about tests or interviews, but never for no reason.

> I get all worked up about nothing, or about something really minor.

> Things I could handle easily in the past seem to really get to me now; I get anxious and upset so easily.

Joe describes his panic reaction as a series of symptoms beginning with a feeling of danger, followed by panic when he cannot determine the cause of the anxiety. He feels a surge of adrenalin and strange sensations, including a fear of dying or going insane. At such times he feels safe only at home because of the unpredictability of the sudden onset of symptoms, particularly those that provoke anxiety. Harold Levinson, M.D., links the anxiety, panic, and phobia symptoms to the "internal state of alarm" that "results when the brain receives scrambled information," attributing the emotions to malfunctions in the cerebellar vestibular system (1986).

The fight-or-flight response is a normal response to stressful stimuli, and its symptoms include shortness of breath, internal chemical changes, increased muscle tension, and circulatory changes. These changes are accompanied by feelings of lightheadedness and fuzzy thinking. When this response occurs in the absence of dangerous stimuli, the sensations are unexplained and can cause us to feel anxious and uncomfortable.

Depression

The medical profession often views depression—and/or an inability to cope productively with stress—as likely causes of any symptoms for which a physiological cause cannot be determined. Thus, psychiatry becomes the dumping ground for those with unexplained illness. Although the fields of psychiatry and psychology are valuable in the treatment of many disorders, indiscriminate referral of those with illnesses of unknown cause is inappropriate.

Depression almost invariably accompanies CFIDS. Because many of the symptoms of depression and CFIDS overlap, it is important to differentiate between depression alone and depression that is a manifestation of CFIDS. The appropriate diagnostic guidelines should be used to make this determination.

Depression may be of the endogenous or exogenous types. In most CFIDS cases it is a combination of the two. Endogenous depression, or depression from within, is thought to have a physical origin, an imbalance in brain chemistry, and may have a genetic basis. The onset of endogenous depression may be abrupt or gradual and is generally unexplained. Exogenous depression (also called reactive depression) is depression "from without" and is attributable to an external event, such as a loss or chronic illness. This type of depression is more common in the general population. In CFIDS, disturbed body chemistry combined with deprivations, losses, changes in lifestyle, and the lack of understanding and empathy of others can produce profound depression. The depression may become more profound with time, as the illness lingers and the hopelessness and helplessness continue. The incidence and severity of the depression may wax and wane, sometimes in rhythm with other CFIDS symptoms.

Symptoms of depression include the following:

feelings of hopelessness, helplessness, and loss of control
    over one's own life
loss of pleasure in life, especially in activities once enjoyed
feelings of worthlessness, self-deprecation, and guilt
inability to concentrate; memory problems
changes in appetite
changes in sleeping patterns (sleeping too much or too
    little; frequent awakenings; early-morning awakening)
feelings of guilt
loss of interest in the outside world
loss of interest in sex
thoughts of suicide, or planning one's suicide

Some CFIDS patients described their feelings of depression:

It comes on me out of nowhere, like I'm suddenly enveloped in a black cloud. It may last a day or two. I hole up in my room; I don't want to talk to anyone. I hate myself, and I'm not fit company. I have no interest in other people or in my normal life activities. I just don't care about anything, least of all myself. It lifts as suddenly as it hit.

When the depression hits, I try to get out of it. Sometimes I can't, but I try. It takes so much effort to be depressed and so much effort to try to get out of it. In the past, when I'd become depressed, it was situationally caused. This is different.

Depression is different from anxiety . . . . Depression is more debilitating.

Even when I have good days, and I feel on top of the world, later it's back down again, sometimes worse than before. Other times it's not as bad and I can come out of it again.

I have reached the point of planning my suicide. I realize that something must be done but I don't have the energy to do anything. I can't work, can't pay my bills or keep my personal life going. This is very difficult for someone who has always done everything, who carried twenty-one or twenty-two semester hours per semester and graduated summa cum laude.

I feel crazy and out of control, and I really don't give a shit about anything. Life just seems so hopeless.

Others may react strangely to our depression, often not understanding that it is beyond voluntary control, that we cannot simply think positively and snap ourselves out of it. Their attempts to cheer us up may backfire by causing us to feel condescended to and terribly misunderstood.

Depression is not a sign of unworthiness, incompetence, or weakness. It is more profound than the sense of discouragement that is likely to accompany any exacerbation of symptoms. Depression is a serious matter; its severity and debilitating effects must not be minimized. If depression is prolonged, severe in degree and duration, or accompanied by suicidal ideation, treatment should be sought immediately.

Chapter 6

◆

Exacerbations and Remissions

WHEN ASKED WHAT HE THOUGHT about the exacerbation-remission cycle, one patient said, "I'd rather have a Honda."

It's like riding the waves: slowly we climb and climb . . . and then, crash! But the ocean waves are somewhat predictable; they follow a pattern. CFIDS symptoms come and go unpredictably, without any regard for any other plans we may have made. Sometimes we can identify the events or exertions that trigger an exacerbation, and at other times they occur for no apparent reason. We seek to identify a catalyst, both to have something to blame (in the absence of this, we often blame ourselves) and to determine what activities or substances to avoid or minimize in the future. On the other hand, some patients experience a steadier illness course with fewer dramatic fluctuations. There may be periods of relative calm interspersed with crashes, or an overall level course of feeling unwell.

EXACERBATIONS: TRIGGERS

Exacerbations may be triggered by changes of almost any kind—physical, emotional, or environmental. Some of the factors that can precede relapses are:

changes in weather, temperature, barometric pressure,
   altitude, humidity, or general climate

overexertion: periods of intense or increased physical
   activity

emotionally stressful events, such as family problems or
   increased demands at work or elsewhere

allergy season or exposure to allergens or substances to
   which one is sensitive

changes in weather (especially abrupt or severe changes)

changes in diet or water source

pregnancy (which causes remission in some cases)

immunosuppression

other illnesses or infections

surgery

antibiotics

travel, especially by airplane (the reason for this is not
   clear but may involve altitude changes, toxic fumes,
   abrupt changes in climate, or recirculated air in
   planes)

Various PWCs describe exacerbations of symptoms preceded by
triggering events:

I've always been the family caretaker, the peacekeeper, everyone's confidante. When there's family stress, like relationship
problems between my parents, I get sicker.

I have to be careful, to guard against exhaustion. Reading
about this illness makes me feel morbid and anxious; this focus
worsens the illness. I'm unable to determine an appropriate
activity level. When should I crusade? When should I rest?
What can I handle?

I did real well when I was working full-time and wasn't smoking. I started smoking again about eight months ago, and my
health has deteriorated gradually. There have also been stressful events since then in my personal life: a divorce, a new
relationship, and changes in my work schedule. I think all of
these things that have happened to me have made this decline
happen.

I went for a job interview. I was thinking about how I'd have to organize my life in order to work. Then, at the interview, the room was spinning; they wanted focused answers, concentration. It was a draining experience. When it was over I wanted to go home and collapse, and they wanted me to do an extra test. By then I was totally out of it: the room was spinning, I was exhausted and fatigued. [Before this interview] I had been feeling better and then I realized that a focused, short period of stress...could quickly catapult me into that dead-ened zone. Just because I had something stressful for a day or two, I was wiped out. It took several days at least before I was back to where I was before I started the whole thing.

Having been advised to resume normal activity levels by a doctor who was unable to diagnose his problem, Bill says:

I took his advice, got out of bed, and went back to the office. It was very poor advice; I got worse again. I was not ready to go back to the office. I'm self-employed, which makes me tend to work harder. I probably would have been better off in bed.

UNPREDICTABLE EXACERBATIONS

Acceptance is undone by nasty surprises.
Cheri Register, *Living with Chronic Illness*

In the preceding cases, the triggers were known or suspected. At other times, the exacerbation may occur for no apparent reason.

Toni Jeffreys wrote in *The Mile-High Staircase*:

I sank down rather less gracefully than a dying duck .... Once again I was hauled up those stairs to bed. I was quite hysterical. Hysterical with the horror of finding myself back in the nightmare. Every cell was crying out. My body was leaden. My head was in agony. I cried and screamed with what little strength there was left. And then I lay staring at the familiar hateful bedroom wall ....

The unthinkable had happened. Again. Every cell in the body, in the brain, was once again crying. Crying out for want of some absolutely necessary chemical, or else suffused with the wrong ones. I was by then battling with the deepest depression. Was I to spend yet another year feeling not dead/not alive? Was there no end to it?...I was vulnerable, vulnerable. (pp. 84, 129).

PWCs describe unpredicted and unwelcome exacerbations:

Some days I feel really good and calm and relaxed; things are going well and the world is nice and rosy. There are other days, the downers, when I don't want to put forth any energy or mess with anything; I just want to feel good.

Every morning I wake up and think, "I wonder how I'm going to feel today."

It's a crapshoot. When will I feel worse and when better? I can't figure it out. As the little girl next door used to say, in response to a question for which she didn't have an answer, "I can't know."

This is such an up-and-down thing; you feel like you're getting better and you feel like you can handle it, and then— Boom! Problems again, you start from scratch again, you lose hope again. How many times can you go on the roller coaster?

Warning signs

Although relapses are usually unpredictable, some PWCs have discovered a particular exacerbation-remission cycle. For example, Bill reports attacks every two to three weeks that last four or five days. Others report a six-week cycle: six "up" weeks followed by six "down" weeks. For some the cycle is not consistent, but preceding the exacerbations they notice warning signs such as fatigue, headache, paleness, muscle aches, visual disturbance, food cravings, or slowed speech, movement, and reactions. Other people may notice these changes before the PWC is aware of them. One of Sara's friends can tell in the first few seconds of a telephone conversation that Sara is having a "tired" or "down" day, and other CFIDS patients report the awareness of people close to them of signs of symptom fluctuations.

I am often surprised when my husband says, "Your speech and movements are slowing down. Do you need to rest?" Most of the time he's correct; I do need to stop and rest and may be starting an exacerbation—but he saw the signs before I did. At other times I am aware of vague warnings: mild muscle aches, fatigue, or equilibrium difficulties. The sooner I pay attention to my body's request for a time-out, the less severe the relapse is likely to be, although sometimes it doesn't seem to matter what I do or how soon I do it. The sick and tired feelings come back full force, and I again feel victimized by a mysterious force outside my control.

Emotional fallout

It's tempting to assign blame when exacerbations occur. We search for a cause or a scapegoat, but sometimes there is none to be found, and we end up blaming ourselves. "It is quite common to feel ashamed or guilty when the illness worsens," writes Cheri Register about illness cycles. "Most of us would rather believe that mind has authority over matter, if we can only learn how to enforce it." So we heap the self-blame on top of the devastating disappointment of the crash, creating a bitter stew of fear, guilt, betrayal, and helplessness. Our feelings run the gamut from hope to desperation, from guilt to anger, as our lives bounce between harmony and discord.

AH! REMISSIONS

To feel good again is exciting—to feel that the virus, or whatever it is, has gone away forever or disappeared into hiding. It feels so good to feel good! Still, the doubt lingers: how long will this last? We learn to savor the moment, pushing back our fears of plummeting again, entering a period of tentative optimism. We're ever-cautious, alert for signs that the grace period is over and it's time to be miserably sick again.

We hope the remission is permanent; the disease is over. We don't ever want to return to that other state. During a remission I wrote in my journal:

> The exacerbation is a black hole. I'm acutely aware of every second—difficult, dark, empty, painful. Then when the sun breaks through, the pain becomes a blur. I wonder where I've been all that time, where my self has been. I am so grateful to have the kind of day that was once only average. An almost-normal day reminds me that I am still myself.

Another excerpt, different remission:

> Oh shit, I'm feeling better and getting hopeful again. Maybe I'm really getting over this—but I've thought that before and then crashed. Each time, like now, I get scared. Each crash is more difficult than the one before it. I love to feel like this, my spunky, smart-ass self again. Now it's scary to feel this good. However, I sure know how to appreciate the value of feeling normal, feeling good, which I used to take for granted. Do I dare believe I'm getting well, or am I just buoyed up by this temporary semi-security, waiting for a fall?

The freshness and energy of remission are invigorating. Hope is rekindled; life matters again. We get back in touch with the pleasant sensations of living and are able to appreciate beauty. We are able to see beyond our own boundaries.

Just as exacerbation is a self-centered event, remission represents an opening of the self to others and to the environment. One hopeful sign for me is becoming aware of the world around me and wanting to do things for others. One day as I gradually awakened from a depressing relapse, I discovered with joy an impulse to get a balloon bouquet for my husband for no apparent reason other than to share my good feelings with him. It was a hopeful time—at best, I was getting better; at worst, I'd feel good for a finite period of time. Either way, I felt wonderful.

In remission I am able to laugh again. I listen to music again, and sing along (much to the dismay of others around me, who may prefer my exacerbations to my musical entertainment). I can balance my outward-and inward-orientations; self-esteem soars. I feel good about others because I am able to feel good about myself.

While feeling better, we want to forget that the "pardon" is temporary, but the fear lingers. Ever aware of the possibility of relapse, we try to pace ourselves to ward off the lurking, unpredictable menace.

When feeling better we tend to overdo, thinking that feeling okay grants us permission to make up for lost time. Such behavior leads to an excessive amount of activity that may put us back in bed. Of course, being careful doesn't guarantee indefinite postponement of an exacerbation, but at least it doesn't invite one. A moderate activity level is difficult to achieve, and the temptation to overdo is enormous.

Exacerbations inevitably occur, despite self-care and preventive measures. The crash produces the familiar sense of defeat and discouragement, and grueling self-questioning about what we've done wrong, what we've done to deserve *this*. Still, as pleasure-seeking human beings, we want to go for it; we try to enjoy the good times while remaining ever-cautious, almost superstitious.

Andy Rooney wrote in a piece entitled "The Flu": "It's difficult to remember how you felt when you were well while you're sick; and difficult to recall how you felt when you were sick when you're well." When I'm feeling better, I can remember feeling lousy, but I can't recapture the true misery and pain of the awful times. Perhaps that's best. We have built-in mechanisms for forgetting pain. (Otherwise everyone would be an only child.) But when the misery returns, the memory is quickly rekindled: back in the black hole, hoping for another reprieve.

Chapter 7

$\blacklozenge$

In Search of a Cause

THE IMMUNE SYSTEM: A CRASH COURSE

In an important sense, the immune system is far
greater than the sum of its parts.
Mizel and Jaret, *The Human Immune Systems:*
The New Frontier in Medicine

Immunology is a relatively new field of medicine; many doctors
practicing today didn't even study it in medical school. In the
past twenty years progress in technology has allowed us to study
the immune system, which is far more complex and important
than previously imagined. It had been believed that the immune
system was complete in and of itself, with little connection to
other body systems. This notion has proven false. The immune
system is integrated with all other bodily systems and our understanding of its functioning is still rudimentary.

The immune system has no central regulating organ, as do
other body systems (e.g., the circulatory system has the heart as
its central organ; the respiratory system, the lungs). Its components are located throughout the body. Communication takes
place among immune cells and between the immune system
and other organs.

The primary function of the immune system is to be sensitive to invaders, to distinguish between "self" and "nonself."

Anything foreign to the body is "nonself": a potential enemy, called an *antigen*. The immune system is capable of identifying a tremendous number of different antigens. Once an enemy is recognized, a complex process is set in motion.

Functioning of the immune system

The following is a simplified explanation of a very powerful and complex process by which our bodies defend themselves against invasion.

There are three basic types of immune cells involved: *phagocytes* (white blood cells, the body's scavengers or garbage collectors which, Pacman-like, gobble up invaders) and the *T-* and *B-cells*, which are types of lymphocytes. (B-cells mature in the bone marrow, T-cells in the thymus gland.) Lymph nodes, the "organs" of the immune system, are small lumps of glandular tissue along lymph channels, through which lymphocytes flow. Lymph nodes are found throughout the body: in the throat area below the tonsils, in the armpits and groin, behind the knees, in many joints, at the base of the lungs, and in the abdomen.

Phagocytes find and attempt to destroy foreign substances ingested from the environment, such as chemical toxins and pollutants. If enemy cells are multiplying so fast that the phagocytes can't keep up with them, they can sound an alarm to alert the rest of the troops. When viruses, bacteria, protozoa, fungi, and other organic invaders attack the body, a complex battle ensues.

The players

Antigens: Substances recognized by the immune system as "nonself," triggering a complex immune response. In the example following these definitions, the antigen is a virus.

Viruses: The invaders—bundles of genetic material in search of a home where they can find host cells in which to thrive and reproduce. A virus that is too successful will sabotage its own life by killing its host. If it is just successful enough, it will coexist with us so that we will survive and serve its needs.

Macrophages: One type of circulating phagocyte that roves the body on the lookout for invaders, which they attempt to gobble up, while summoning additional help from helper T-cells.

Helper T-cells: The stars of the team that orchestrate the battle. Helper T-cells circulate throughout body tissues, serving as sentries. When T-cells become aware of an enemy invasion, they begin to multiply and also alert the spleen and lymph nodes to encourage the production of other immune cells by means of *lymphokine* (immune system "communicator chemicals") signals. Each of the many varieties of helper T-cells is programmed to recognize a specific enemy.

Killer T-cells: Cells summoned by the helper T-cells that act as their name implies: they rush to the site of the invasion and attempt to kill the invaders.

B-cells: Munitions factories in the spleen or lymph nodes. Arriving helper T-cells stimulate production of B-cells, which produce antibodies designed specifically for the type of invader.

Antibodies: Protein molecules produced by B-cells that are designed specifically to combat particular invaders. Antibodies rush to the war zone to neutralize or destroy enemy cells.

Suppressor T-cells: After the invaders have been conquered, the suppressor T-cells call off the attack by stopping the B- and T-cell activity.

Memory cells: These circulate in the body with a memory of a previous attacker so that a subsequent attack by the same type of enemy can be more easily conquered, even many years later. Vaccines stimulate production of memory cells. When antibodies are produced to such substances as pollens or cat dander, we are said to be allergic to these things.

The process

The process of a viral attack begins with the virus entering the body. Its presence is noticed by macrophages, which attempt to destroy it. The macrophages call for helper T-cells, which become active and multiply. Specific killer T- and B-cells are produced to launch an attack on the invader. The B-cells produce antibodies against the invader. Since some of the invading viral cells have infiltrated host cells, killer T's attempt to kill the invaded cells. Antibodies then neutralize the viruses by attaching to them (to prevent them from invading other cells) and producing substances intended to poison the infected cells. After the infection has been halted, other T-cells call off the battle, shutting off the immune response. Memory cells memorize the chemical identities of the conquered attackers so they can recognize them should they reattack in the future. Although this is the basic program by which the immune system is believed to fight off infection, the process is actually much more complex, and much of it is not currently understood. (*Note:* This summary is based in part on a section of Peter Jaret's excellent article "The Wars Within," *National Geographic,* June 1986.)

Immunological research has led to a knowledge of protein substances called lymphokines, the immune messengers that cause the production of such symptoms as fever and inflammation, indicating that the immune system is at war with an invader. Some lymphokines are thought to be able to kill enemy cells directly, such as some cancer cells. Examples of lymphokines are interleukins (ILs), B-cell growth factor, B-cell differentiation factor, and the interferons. Lymphokines are now recognized as extremely important parts of the immune response, and they are being used in the treatment of cancer and other diseases. Some researchers feel that a better understanding of lymphokine functioning and identification of currently unknown lympyhokines will provide the keys for understanding and treating immune problems as well as some psychiatric disorders that may be immune-related.

Because CFIDS involves disregulation of the immune system, many of its symptoms may be caused by an immune imbalance, specifically in levels of various lymphokines. When the immune system is constantly turned on, it reacts to all types of substances perceived as "nonself," producing the various discomforts of CFIDS. (Keep in mind that our symptoms may be caused by our bodies' *reactions* to particular agents, such as viruses, rather than by the direct action of those agents.)

IMMUNE DYSFUNCTION

When the immune system is not functioning perfectly a number of problems may develop, some apparent and others subtle. Immune dysfunction is probably a contributory factor in many currently unexplained illnesses. Improper immune functioning occurs when the immune system underreacts, overreacts, or reacts inappropriately to an invader. When it reacts appropriately, we are able to fight off, or resist, infection. When the immune system's attempts are inadequate, illness is the result. We are constantly exposed to many antigens; only when the antigens "win" do we get sick.

The interaction of helper and suppressor T-cells is the on-off switch of the immune system. The ratio of helper to suppressor T-cells is normally 2:1 or 3:1. The balance between them is critical to proper immune response and functioning. During and following illness, this ratio varies.

In **autoimmune disorders,** the immune system has lost its ability to distinguish between "self" and "nonself," and the body attacks its own tissue as if it were an antigen (enemy). In the process healthy cells are attacked and destroyed. Multiple sclerosis, rheumatoid arthritis, some forms of thyroid disease, and systemic lupus erythematosus are considered autoimmune disorders. The incidence of autoimmune diseases is thought to be higher in women, possibly due to hormonal factors or immune systems that respond more aggressively to invaders.

A state of **immunosuppression** allows enemy cells, such as viruses, to reproduce actively. The situation may be a "stand-off" in which the immune system is unable to rid the body of invaders and keeps them somewhat in check. When the immune system is rallying, symptoms subside. When the disruptive agent becomes stronger, symptoms increase. Neither side is able to sustain a victory and end the war. As the war continues, the infectious agent retains a degree of control; if the agent "lost" it would be killed. If the agent "won" it would kill the patient, thus destroying itself. So it is to the invader's advantage to stay in control by using the host but not killing it. In the process, it attempts to disrupt the host's functioning in ways that will make the invader's life happier—and the host's life more miserable.

Immune dysfunction can be caused by a variety of factors. Primary immune deficiencies (those that are congenital, or present from birth) may not become apparent until later in life when exposure to certain antigens creates symptoms. Secondary immune deficiencies are acquired; they develop as a result of nongenetic factors such as nutrition, age, amount of sleep, surgery and general anesthesia, infections, injury, certain drugs, emotional state, hormonal imbalance, stress level, and exposure to various environmental toxins and allergens. Such deficiencies may be transient; for example, when an infection has been successfully resolved or when exposure to a toxin is discontinued, the deficiency may also resolve.

Negative emotional states, such as loneliness and depression, can impair immunity to a significant degree because of alterations of neuroendocrine function (or the connections between the brain and the glandular system). Intense and/or prolonged stress adversely affects immune functioning. Constant stress response (the fight-or-flight reaction) and the negative emotions affect hormonal, neural, and endocrine function, which in turn cause the immune system to function less efficiently. Conversely, positive emotions and a hopeful outlook are believed to enhance immune functioning.

When the immune system is out of balance, some parts become overactive and others underactive. The problem is not that the immune system isn't reacting *strongly* enough but that it's reacting inappropriately. The signals being sent between the parts of the immune system, and between the immune system and the rest of the body, may be distorted, creating malfunctions in the entire body system. Excessive, futile attention focused on a benign invader (such as pollen) while a more significant threat is ignored is analogous to an individual shooting bullets at a harmless fly while ignoring a burglar who is looting the contents of the house.

So far there has been a lack of consistency in findings regarding immune dysfunction in CFIDS as well as great difficulty in correlating measurable abnormalities with the patient's symptoms. Immune abnormalities are a piece of the CFIDS puzzle, but it is still not known whether the abnormalities are a cause or effect (or both) of the illness. Techniques for measuring immune function are fairly rudimentary and we are unable to measure the strength of an individual's immune system. We are able to measure certain types of immune functioning but these measurements are not comprehensive (or generalizable) and are often inaccurate.

A landmark medical journal article entitled "Phenotypic and Functional Deficiency of Natural Killer Cells in Patients with Chronic Fatigue Syndrome" reported abnormal activity and ratios of natural killer cells, a "first line of defense in animals against viral infections." The researchers were not able to determine whether this aberration was a cause or effect of CFIDS but it was significant in that it was the first documented immune abnormality. (Caliguiri et al., 1987). Since that time other immune abnormalities have been noted in PWCs (as described in Chapter 4) but, unfortunately, such abnormalities are difficult to test for, test results are inconsistent, and findings vary among patients. But the types of abnormalities found in PWCs yield insight into the mechanisms involved in CFIDS and offer additional treatment options.

The essential question, then, is not simply, "What goes wrong with the immune system that makes us sick?" or "What is the virus or other causative agent that makes us sick?" but the more complex question, "How do these various factors interact to make us sick?" The cause(s) and contributing factors are likely to include the following:

Viruses

Viruses are submicroscopic, protein-covered bundles of genetic material containing blueprints for self-reproduction. Viruses are covered with a capsid, or coat, and/or a special envelope, which they use to attach to the cells they subsequently enter. In fact, many antiviral drugs work by damaging or destroying these coats so that attachment cannot take place. Unlike bacteria, which are living organisms, viruses are neither alive nor dead. Incapable of reproduction on their own, they search for hosts whose cells they can invade to accomplish this purpose. They invade our cells (like checking into a motel) and give genetic orders, turning our cells into virus factories. Their offspring burst forth, destroying the previously invaded cell and seeking out new healthy cells for their continued reproduction. These tiny, elusive viruses are capable of hiding, mutating, and combining. There are many types of viruses (probably hundreds of thousands), only some of which have been identified. Because viruses are adept at escaping detection, viral illnesses are often diagnosed on the basis of symptoms and by exclusion of other possible illnesses. We can guess about them based on the damage they do, and we identify them based on the antibodies produced in reaction to their presence. Viruses are capable of altering their identity by mutating.

Many viruses can remain in latent (nonreproducing) form in our bodies for long periods of time without producing symptoms. Viral agents that may produce latent (inactive) infections include herpes simplex, herpes zoster, cytomegalovirus (CMV), human herpesvirus Type 6 (HHV-6), and retroviruses. Many viruses are capable of producing chronic illnesses by alternating dormant and active (replication) phases. Their versatility allows viruses to exist in an active, dormant, or low-level state, producing varied immune reactions in our bodies. Factors that facilitate reactivation of latent viruses include infections (for example, infection with one virus may trigger activation of another dormant virus), exposure to certain chemicals (allergens, toxins, immunosuppressive drugs), fever, corticosteroids, physical or emotional stress, ultraviolet light, and local trauma.

Certain viral disorders are believed to be linked with disorders elsewhere in the body, for example in the nervous system, the endocrine system, and the immune system. Future research will likely reveal the nature of these links.

Several viruses are being studied to determine their possible roles in CFIDS. They fall into various classes. Adenoviruses can infect cells and can persist for long periods of time. They can reproduce slowly but consistently, producing low-grade infections. Slow viruses have long incubation periods and can cause persistent disease (often neurological) after being in the body for a long period of time. Viruses in the herpes class demonstrate a particular ability to remain latent for long periods of time. Herpesvirus infections include cold sores, herpes encephalitis, influenza-type illness, chicken pox and shingles (both caused by the varicella virus), cytomegalovirus-related illness (which occurs mainly in fetuses and babies, but which can also produce a mono-like illness), and mononucleosis. Certain herpes viruses are believed to play a role in some forms of cancer.

The Epstein-Barr virus (EBV) is a herpes virus that infects virtually everyone; 90–95% of the adult population have antibodies to it, meaning that they have been infected at some time during their lives (in many cases, without obvious symptoms). Once the virus has infected an individual, it persists for life, generally remaining inactive following the initial exposure, probably because we've developed enough antibodies to suppress the virus but not kill it. EBV infections in children are generally asymptomatic. Young adults initially exposed to it may develop mononucleosis, which typically lasts about six weeks, although symptoms may persist for months. Reports of chronic mononucleosis (mono that doesn't clear up after six weeks to six months) have been documented. EBV may play a role in CFIDS, although in most cases not a causative one. Chronic mononucleosis has never been known to appear in epidemic form. In CFIDS and other illnesses, a weakened immune system may allow replication of EBV and other previously dormant viruses. It is also possible that we are faced with a new strain of the EB virus in CFIDS.

Human herpesvirus Type 6 (HHV-6), previously known as HBLV, has been another suspect in the recent outbreaks of CFIDS. Discovered in 1986 by researchers at the National Cancer Institute, HHV-6 is a latent virus; like EBV, it can remain dormant in the body for long periods of time and is subject to reactivation by various factors. The presence of

HHV-6 in large numbers of CFIDS patients may indicate a causal role, but is more likely a signal of immune dysfunction. Its prevalence in the normal population has not been ascertained; many of those infected show no symptoms.

Other viruses that may play a role in causation and/or symptom production are cytomegalovirus, which causes symptoms similar to those caused by EBV, notably neurological ones, coxsackie virus, herpes zoster (which causes chicken pox and shingles and remains dormant in the nerve cells thereafter), and other herpesviruses, such as herpes simplex I and II (formerly referred to as oral and genital herpes). All of these viruses tend to become more active when the human host is under increased stress.

Byron Hyde, M.D., of Canada speculates that CFIDS, or ME (myalgic encephalomyelitis) as it is called there, is caused by an enterovirus (a category of viruses that includes Coxsackie and polio). There is some speculation that CFIDS is another form of poliomyelitis or is caused by a nonpolio enterovirus—or that enteroviruses do not play a causal role but are reactivated by immune disregulation, as are the herpesviruses, for example.

A more recent suspect is a retrovirus—possibly human T-Lymphotrophic Virus Type 2 (HTLV-2). Retroviruses contain an enzyme called reverse transcriptase that allows them to reverse the order of genetic information processing—hence their name. Retroviruses have been implicated in such illnesses as AIDS, a rare type of leukemia, and certain forms of cancer. Research findings by Dr. Elaine DeFreitas at the Wistar Institute, in conjunction with Drs. Bell and Cheney and other researchers, were presented at the Eleventh International Congress of Neuropathology in Kyoto, Japan, in September 1990. In a large percentage of the small number of cases studied they reported the presence of certain viral sequences that resemble HTLV-2 but which also might be a new, previously undiscovered retrovirus that shares a common gene sequence with HTLV-2. It is also possible that a retrovirus interacts with other viruses to cause CFIDS.

Another retroviral suspect is spumavirus, a virus whose cultured cells appear clumped and foamy, previously known to infect only animals and never before linked to human disease. Tests have revealed this type of virus to be present in many of the PWCs tested, but its role in CFIDS, as reported by such researchers as Drs. Behan, DeFreitas, Grossberg, and Martin, is unclear. Spumavirus has been cultured in about half of the PWCs studied in preliminary tests, and it may be that those with evidence of encephalopathy are most likely to test positive.

The significance of these early studies is the finding of nonubiquitous viruses in PWCs, according to Dr. DeFreitas, who believes that retroviruses are suggested as causal agents because they are neurotropic (they live in the brain and other parts of the central nervous sustem) and because retroviruses are associated with immune dysfunction (November 1991). However, to make any causal assumptions about these preliminary findings would be premature. The possibility of retroviral involvement in CFIDS is a first significant step in what will doubtless be a lengthy research process which may yield a breakthrough—or another blind alley. Such findings have served the important function of alerting the medical profession and the media to the existent seriousness of CFIDS.

We don't know whether CFIDS is virally caused. CFIDS acts like a viral illness: it waxes and wanes and produces a dazzling array of symptoms that vary over time. CFIDS patients often have high levels of anti-viral antibodies that are assumed to indicate viral activation. In our attempts to determine viral involvement in CFIDS, we operate under many handicaps. We are unable to measure viral activity directly, unable to measure antibodies to many viruses, and we don't even know how many varieties of viruses actually exist. In future study, molecular biology will allow us to gain a better understanding of viruses and their involvement in CFIDS.

A virus may be only one of the causal or triggering agents. Nonviral triggering factors that interfere with immune functioning may allow viruses to move from dormant to active states so that viral activation is an effect, rather than a cause, of CFIDS. The cause may turn out to be a newly discovered virus, a more virulent strain of a known virus, a recombinant virus, a faulty immune system reacting inappropriately to a "normal" virus, all of the above—or none of the above. And, of course, CFIDS may be an umbrella term for a number of different but similar illnesses with various causative factors. Even if the cause of CFIDS is viral, there may be no one particular virus that is causal in all cases.

And if a virus or viruses are implicated, what to do? Detection, the first step, is very difficult. Treatment, the next step, is also difficult. Only one virus, smallpox, is believed to be completely eradicated. There are vaccines for a few viral illnesses: polio, rubella, hepatitis B, and some strains of influenza virus. Another approach to treatment is aimed at increasing immune effectiveness: immune-enhancing drugs are currently used for treating CFIDS and new ones are being developed and tested.

Genetic predisposition

> My immune system isn't what it used to be, and it never was.
>
> *Excerpt from my journal*

Many PWCs report medical histories indicative of long-term low-level immune dysfunction. The following comments are fairly typical:

> I've always thought of myself as a healthy person, but over the years I've had numerous infections and problems with fatigue. But until now I've always recovered uneventfully.

> I've had something in my system all my life; periodically, it flares up. I've had diphtheria three times, Legionnaire's disease, viral pneumonia twice, and cancer. I get sick after stressful events.

> I've had low body temperature all my life, and I've always needed lots of rest.

> I had asthma as a child, measles three times, pneumonia during my third pregnancy, sinus trouble, hepatitis, Legionnaire's disease . . . . But I've always been active and considered myself

healthy. Then, in 1985, I slowed down more and more, stopped ice-skating and running, dropped the aerobics classes I was teaching, one at a time. I felt like a balloon that lost its air.

I had mono when I was 36 [present age 53]. I've had a history of colds, throat problems, allergies. I had rheumatic fever as a child. I've had low stamina all my life. I've always gotten motion sickness and have a tendency to faint.

My immune system has never worked right.

I've had frequent infections all my life, but I've always recovered from them—until this one.

One patient, a retired university professor, speculated that those most prone to get CFIDS have a history of such illnesses as cradle cap, eczema, asthma and other bronchial problems, whooping cough, chicken pox, rubella, measles, allergies, depression, and viral illness, with periodic illnesses and periods of "not feeling well" throughout their lives, interspersed with times of relatively normal functioning. He believes that such a history, combined with the stress of Type A behavior and a busy lifestyle, contributes strongly to the development of CFIDS. Many patient interviews strengthen this impression, but it is dangerous to draw conclusions from such sketchy data.

Such histories suggest that an incompetent immune system, either genetic or acquired, may contribute to the development of CFIDS in susceptible individuals. However, many other PWCs report a history of good health, rarely missing school or work, with little tendency to get colds or flu.

Environment

> ... [T]oo many major American industries dig up the good things out of the earth, spit out what they can't use and produce poisonous waste by-products that are eventually going to kill the land and then us .... While the leaders of government everywhere are worrying about the Big Bomb, mankind everywhere is poisoning the ground and the waters we depend on for life.
>
> Andy Rooney, *The Dead Land*

Hippocrates stressed the importance of viewing the human body within its context—its geography, climate, diet, and so on. Our environment is a dangerous place to live. We are subjected to pollutants in the air we breathe, additives in our food, and contaminants in our drinking water. We ingest harmful chemicals in startling amounts daily. We are poisoning ourselves slowly with substances whose potential damage we can only estimate. The so-called safe amounts of these chemicals are mere guesses, their synergistic effects are totally unknown. Government regulations are inadequate and poorly enforced. In recent years the number of new chemicals introduced into our bodies has increased dramatically, until our bodies are like chemical processing plants that are heavily and unreasonably taxed, affecting all levels of functioning. In the name of progress we have created compounds that are both helpful and harmful, and the immune system bears the brunt of their assault. Just a few of the culprits found in air, soil, and water are pesticides (insecticides and herbicides such as chlordane), food additives (e.g., preservatives; flavoring and coloring agents; steroids, veterinary medicines, and antibiotics in meat and poultry; waxes; thickening agents; emulsifiers), and air pollutants (e.g., sulfur dioxide).

Anyone would refuse a cocktail made of arsenic, aldicarb (a pesticide), vinyl chloride (used in making plastic), polychlorinated biphenyls (PCBs), hazardous industrial solvents, radioactive wastes, and heavy metals (such as chromium, lead, and cadmium)—yet we ingest these substances frequently. They may affect our immune systems adversely, but we fool ourselves with a game called, "What I can't see can't hurt me."

In "The Poisons Within," a six-part series which appeared in *The Arizona Republic*, Mike Masterson, investigative team leader wrote:

> Americans are consuming an unprecedented number of hazardous chemicals in their food, water, and air. Some are becoming ill and dying from this relatively new threat, but no one knows the extent of the long-term effects. (January 29, 1989)

Scientists are concerned that sustained low-level exposure to many different types of manufactured chemicals will damage *immune or neurological functions* and elevate cancer rates over the coming decades. (January 29, 1989) [italics added]

Ground water in at least portions of every state is contaminated with cancer-causing pesticides, solvents or other hazardous chemicals. New contamination sites are being discovered every year. (January 31, 1989)

The federal agencies that once told Americans they could ingest small amounts of the pesticide DDT [now banned for its toxicity] without fear today assure them it is all right to ingest minuscule levels of many pesticides that have yet to be thoroughly tested. (February 1, 1989)

Some pesticide residues, or metabolites, are present in almost all American adults. One 1987 study showed evidence of three potent pesticides in 72 percent of the urine samples taken from 28,000 people in 64 communities. (February 1, 1989)

Federally permissible traces of various pesticides and drugs exist in much of the meat and poultry that Americans consume, resulting in a cumulative effect on the body when they combine with other chemicals in fruits, vegetables and water. (February 3, 1989)

Each month many new chemicals are registered, adding to the existing risks. "Americans routinely ingest thousands of these man-made chemicals created, ironically, to enhance the quality of life. Many compounds remain in the body for years." (January 29, 1989). Many banned substances continue to be used either in the U.S. or in countries from which we import food.

The toll on human life is gradual and subtle, but alarming. Even if we were to begin an aggressive clean-up program on a national level, much of the damage cannot be undone because many of these dangerous substances are stored indefinitely in adipose tissue (fat), the cumulative and synergistic (combined) effects are unknown, and irreversible genetic changes may have already taken place. In addition, a comprehensive program to make dramatic changes in our use of these chemicals would be politically unpopular because of its astronomical cost. Our government is more responsive to market pressures than to social welfare; because the use of harmful chemicals is economically profitable its impact on health is almost ignored. The long-term damage to our bodies cannot be assessed but these dangerous substances are believed to cause immune and nervous system disorders. Unless we make massive clean-up efforts a priority, the damage will continue to compound.

Disease symptoms related to the ingestion of toxic substances in the workplace show up in many occupations. For example, daily exposure to solvents has produced cognitive dysfunction, aggressiveness, mental fatigue, and disturbances in social relationships (Orbaek and Lindgren, 1988, pp. 37, 43). Office personnel in large, sealed buildings are subject to increased exposure to viruses and bacteria as the air endlessly recirculates. Daniel Peterson, M.D., commented on the closed-building phenomenon in relation to the CFIDS outbreak in Lake Tahoe, stating that the incidence of CFIDS in local schools with poor air exchange had been significantly greater than its incidence in schools with better air circulation (May 1991). However, the possible connection between closed buildings and CFIDS has not been studied systematically. Another unknown is the effect of electromagnetic pollution: we are subjected to electromagnetic fields created by power stations, power lines, and home appliances daily, but little research regarding their effects has been done.

Environmental pollution and illness, immune dysfunction, and CFIDS may be inextricably related.

Stress

Stress is natural and necessary. In and of itself stress is not bad, it is simply continual adaptation to demands from without and within. In a positive sense, stress is the force that urges us forward, allowing growth and progress. Even positive events—a promotion at work or a new addition to the family—are stressful in that adaptation is required. When stressors are numerous, severe, and/or constant, or when we fail to adapt successfully, the result of stress can be bodily damage. Sources of stress are everywhere in our lives: too much or too little activity, the demands of families and employers, responsibilities, excessive noise and environmental pollution, and so on.

The amount and nature of the stressors and our individual ability to adapt successfully determine the toll stress will take. If we neglect self-care (sufficient sleep, moderate exercise, relaxation, and adequate diet) and constantly push to get ahead, our health will be affected. Our society doesn't regard self-care as a priority. To push harder as stressors accumulate is the norm; to pull back and rest as needed is frowned upon. Often we neglect ourselves and our needs because we're on autopilot, putting out lots of time and energy as we're programmed to do, and not caring for ourselves because the notion of self-care may not occur to us, because we may be unaware of its importance. Many of us live in a state of constant tension and anxiety. Stress activates the fight-or-flight response, a protective process in which bodily changes take place and numerous chemicals are released. Some of these chemicals are hormones that inhibit adequate functioning of the immune system. As the body continually taps its resources for coping with stress, certain chemicals become depleted and exhaustion may set in, rendering us susceptible to illness. In the face of continuing challenges we continue to push (rather than to rest as our bodies urge us to do) and our self-neglect compounds the problem. We are essentially drawing from an account which has dipped deeply into credit reserve.

The total stress load on an individual consists of both inner and outer stressors: major life changes and personal crises (identity crises, relationship problems, low self-esteem, disappointments). Unmet needs, challenging events, and the ongoing daily grind contribute to the total load. Unrelenting stress or a series of sudden highly stressful events is taxing even to the strong and hardy.

Many PWCs have described stressful events that preceded the onset of illness: death of loved ones, divorce or breakup of significant relationships, other illnesses (their own, or those of family members or close friends), career or job changes, health problems including illness and surgery, financial problems, moves to different geographical areas, and other individual or family crises. Many stressful events involve some type of loss, and the average number of major stressors reported in a survey of Phoenix PWCs was 3.2 per person in the eighteen months preceding the onset of CFIDS. In addition to these events the majority reported highly active, busy lifestyles, which presented chronic stressors: rapid life changes at the individual and societal levels, economic instability, changing roles, anxieties about spiritual and existential concerns, various life dissatisfactions, time pressures, lack of social structure, and difficulty relaxing.

Many of us have taken on a number of professional and personal roles: we may work several jobs and balance hectic schedules. Recent years have brought a dazzlingly accelerated rate of technological change. Keeping up with the fast pace of life and barrages of sensory input can be overwhelming. We live a crazy lifestyle in which denial of personal needs is considered heroic. We travel widely, diet frequently, intersperse dieting with junk food pig-outs, try to force rapid recovery after surgery or illness, ignore the problems and symptoms that are trying to give us messages about our needs, and spend so much time "taking care of business" that we neglect to take care of ourselves.

One PWC, a former actress, says:

> You put a car in a garage and it will last a lot longer than if you put it in a grand prix all the time. It's going to get worn out; my immune system is worn out. My body is a very important vehicle and I've abused it by overachieving, always being on the go without sufficient food or sleep. I had two surgeries, marital problems and a divorce, and then I got this illness.

Yolanda relates her high stress level to graduate school pressures, family responsibilities, divorce, remarriage, and her self-concept as a superwoman who could and should handle these pressures and transitions easily. She admits that she put others' needs before her own and had always had unrealistically high self-expectations. She developed CFIDS in her final year at graduate school and barely made it through finals. Now unable to work, she wonders if she wasted her time and money to prepare for a career she may never attain.

Another PWC states, "I was going to school, caring for my four kids, and building a house. I lost several friends. My parents became ill and died. I'm in the process of adopting two more kids. I don't have time to be ill." And when she developed CFIDS, her illness became another cause of stress.

Once the diagnosis is made, the CFIDS label is an additional stressor, as is the search for treatment. What would have been minor events in the past become more stressful because of the illness: physical or mental activity, travel, chemical exposure, hormonal fluctuations, and any type of family problems. The body becomes exquisitely sensitive even to minor assaults.

Psychoneuroimmunology

Psychoneuroimmunology (PNI) is a newly-emerging field based on age-old wisdom that asserts that all body systems are interrelated—the central nervous system (brain and spinal cord), the mind, the emotions, the immune system, and so on. According to this concept, all illness is psychosomatic, involving the interaction of mind and body (the "mindbody"). The term psychosomatic, however, is commonly used erroneously, as if to mean "all in one's head," suggesting an illness more imagined than real.

Chronic pain or recurrent symptoms may be viewed as the body's signal that stress overload is occurring. The brain takes in stimuli and communicates its messages to the body, and the various body systems communicate with the brain as well. For example, the hypothalamus (which regulates such functions as sleeping, eating, temperature, glandular activity, and the immune system) sends messenger molecules to the endocrine system, which regulates the body's hormones. A malfunctioning portion of the brain can create many effects which we call symptoms.

Psychosocial and environmental events take their toll on the immune system, but the way in which this occurs is not fully understood. In *The Healer Within*, Locke and Colligan discussed the tendrils of nerve tissue from the brain that run through the most important parts of the immune system: the thymus gland, bone marrow, lymph nodes, and spleen. Hormones and neurotransmitters secreted by the brain have an affinity for immune cells. There are active lines of communication between the brain and the immune system, and brain chemicals have both positive and negative influences on immune functioning. The brain–immune system link works both ways; changes in either entity affect the other because they are inextricably bound. Neither controls the other but each influences the other. The links among all body systems present the opportunity for our emotions to influence how well the body is able to defend itself.

Unfortunately, the medical profession as a whole has not embraced the PNI concept and holds fast to the outdated notion of mind-body duality. The number of medical specialties and sub-specialties offer more effective treatment of certain disorders, but also indicates considerable fragmentation, in which the importance of the interconnections between body systems is minimized. This simple cause-and-effect view hampers our understanding of such complex illnesses as CFIDS.

Other suspected causes/contributing factors

Systemic yeast/fungal infection. Because many CFIDS patients have apparent yeast-related problems, yeast overgrowth may be a causal contributor to CFIDS, or vice versa—or both may be attributable to immune dysfunction. Contributing factors to both conditions may include nutritional deficiencies, overuse of antibiotics, extended use of birth control pills, environmental toxins, and emotional stress—all of which are believed to have detrimental effects on immunity.

The fact that anti-yeast medications and diet are helpful to many PWCs does not prove a causal relationship but does indicate that further research is warranted. It is likely that both yeast overgrowth and CFIDS symptoms are the result of disregulation of the immune system.

Vaccines. Routine immunization has obliterated several life-threatening illnesses but may also have negative effects on the immune systems of susceptible individuals. In particular, certain rubella vaccines introduced in 1979 are suspected as CFIDS-causing (or contributing) agents. Vaccines contain attenuated (weakened) viruses to stimulate the production of antibodies so that the individual will not get an active infection if exposed to the virus at a later time. However, the injected viruses, although attenuated, may be transmitted from those vaccinated (usually children) to others who are sufficiently sensitive to react to the virus and become ill.

SELF-RESPONSIBILITY FOR ILLNESS?

> We were all being assaulted now with the verbiage of self-help guerrillas who said gay men had brought AIDS on themselves. "I'm taking a course in miracles," as one Hollywood airhead shared with me on the phone one night. "People pick their own diseases," he said, bragging that his lesions had faded to inconsequence .... But nobody picks his own disease—except, perhaps, the more rabid religions.
> Paul Monette, *Borrowed Time*

> Humans are unwilling to believe that great suffering and disaster can be inflicted without moral justification.
> Rita Mae Brown, *High Hearts*

Some of us have been led to believe that we have "made ourselves sick." Are we responsible for our illness? Is it something we have chosen? A punishment for not living right? A sign of weakness or personal failure? The result of an inadequate spiritual belief system?

And what does it mean that we have remained sick? That we haven't triumphed, conquered? That we're weak rather than strong? That we have failed to learn the right lessons?

In a *New Age Journal* article, Ken and Treya Wilber discussed the downside of New Age spiritual belief systems that blame patients for their illnesses and insist that new, correct attitudes and beliefs are a primary curative force. According to this new way of thinking, we are supposed to "think" or "will" the disease away. Our inability to rid ourselves of illness can become a source of shame and inadequacy. The Wilbers do not view illness as a punishment or life lesson but as an opportunity to make life changes and achieve greater harmony.

"I blame myself for having gotten sick," says Bill, who thinks a medicine he took might have caused CFIDS. "I'm angry at the doctor who prescribed it and at myself for taking it. I haven't gotten over the guilt and I don't know if I ever will." Kyle comments, "I think we create our own realities and our own diseases. I think there are accidents, but I'm wondering if we didn't create those, too." Yolanda says, "I still feel the guilt of wondering if [CFIDS] is my own fault."

Is illness something we bring upon ourselves as a special challenge, a signal of a particular deficiency needing to be grappled with, a sign that we have not handled our emotions properly? Susan Sontag (1977) believes that the punitive notion of disease causation has been long-standing and counterproductive, encouraging the patient to engage in self-blame for having become ill and then for not getting well. These feelings may retard rather than speed healing. In writing about AIDS, Paul Monette lamented the "growing 'empowerment movement,' which tended to start with the assumption that people brought on their own illness," and suggested that developing the proper attitude would allow the virus to "evaporate like a fog" (1988, p. 227).

We have all questioned ourselves similarly. The verdict is: *Not guilty.* To blame ourselves—or anyone—for our illness is not only erroneous, it's destructive. I don't believe that illness is part of a divine plan, that it is our karma, that we somehow chose it and should be able to will it away. I've been through all that, questioning my attitudes, beliefs, and lifestyle. I've wanted to have someone or something to blame (we're conditioned that way), but I've drawn a blank. I am able to identify some factors that contributed to my susceptibility to this illness, but I no longer look for the cause within myself.

Not wanting to be blamed or seen as weak by others because we are ill, we often attempt to minimize the problem.

"Fine!" we reply heartily when asked how we are feeling. "Doing lots better!" It seems, somehow, to be the respectable and expected response. Irrationally, I sometimes feel I've failed to get well; I feel apologetic, ashamed, and incompetent. Even though I know better, such feelings still surface occasionally and I have to remind myself of their irrationality.

Judging ourselves for being ill is self-defeating. It is essential to develop a sensible belief system about illness, preferably one that includes the following concepts:

> Illness is not a test of character strength or a sign of personal deficiency.
>
> Life is not fair.
>
> Bad things do happen to good people. (Conversely, good things happen to bad people!)
>
> Just because I don't know exactly what caused my illness, that doesn't mean I should blame myself—or anyone.
>
> Question: *Why me?* Answer: *Why not me?*
>
> There are some questions to which we don't have, and may never have, answers.
>
> Having participated to some degree in the origins of an illness is not the same as having caused it or being to blame for it.

Illness did not occur in our lives to present a growth opportunity we needed or invited. But since it has happened to us, we can learn from the experience. We can grow in ways we could not have anticipated and find new meaning and goals in life. Taking the illness as a given, something that happened for a number of reasons that have nothing to do with personal volition or worth, we can decide what to make of it—whether to give in to it or to learn from it, whether to neglect or take care of ourselves to maximize our chances of regaining health. We don't have a choice about whether or not to be sick. It's an opportunity to grow, one we can accept or refuse. But we can't go back to the way we were.

PERSONALITY TYPE AS A CAUSE OF ILLNESS?

Many of those diagnosed with CFIDS were once energetic, driven, aggressive, intelligent, perfectionistic, goal-oriented people with busy lifestyles. Phillip Rubin, M.D., said at a Phoenix support group meeting in 1988, "Most of you do in your impaired state more than most people do in their normal state."

Many PWCs fit the "magic caretaker role." In their personal and professional lives they have always taken care of others, often at their own expense. They have felt most comfortable when providing, even sacrificing, for others and they feel a very strong need to "be good." Others depend on them. They are often over-extended. These are the people-pleasers who make such statements as:

I have taken care of other people all my life.

I've always had an overactive conscience.

In my family, I was the peacemaker, the fixer.

I always wanted to be perfect.

Everyone has always relied on me.

My childhood wish was to do everything there is to do.

I feel like I was addicted to stress, to the adrenaline rush. Relax? No, no, no, no! I just wore myself out because I never let up.

I didn't take vacations . . . and I loved what I was doing, even though the hours were long.

For a long time I worked full-time and went to college part-time. I've done that for years and years and years, as well as taking care of everything that was involved with my family.

I've never been accountable just for me. I've been working for a long time now, going to school, raising kids. You make up your mind to do something; you do it. And all of a sudden I couldn't. Nothing had ever stopped me.

I was very self-sufficient, very independent. I didn't need anybody's help.

To assess changes in personality characteristics pre- and post-CFIDS, I administered a checklist of personality traits to 59 PWCs at a meeting of the CFS Association in Phoenix. The changes indicated were dramatic and are consistent with the suspected typical CFIDS profile:

	Pre-Illness	Currently
Outgoing personality	82%	26%
Introverted personality	11	50
Easygoing	47	21
High achiever	87	18
Energetic, always "on the go"	87	18
Competitive	87	8
Perfectionistic	76	21
Assertive	68	26
High self-confidence	63	26
Caretaker of others	84	34
Independent	92	18
Dependent	11	47
Physically fit	63	3
Financially secure	79	32
Have difficulty asking others to meet your needs	53	53
"Yuppie" lifestyle	39	5
Frequent exercise: vigorous	37	5
Frequent exercise: mild	45	21

Note: It is not known whether PWCs in this group are a representative sample of all PWCs, or if they are those most likely to have pursued a diagnosis, seen multiple doctors, joined support groups, and volunteered for studies, thus skewing (altering) the results. More passive PWCs may remain undiagnosed, see fewer doctors, and be less likely to become active in organizations and studies.

Kenneth Pelletier (1977) views the "Type A" person as competitive, driven, hostile, impatient, accomplishment-oriented, aggressive, extroverted, and internally insecure. The Type A person feels a constant sense of time urgency, often places great emphasis on monetary success, is easily aroused, has a difficult time relaxing, and focuses single-mindedly on present achievements rather than on the overall view of life. The Type B person feels less time urgency, values leisure time and uses it without guilt, is more likely to be committed to meaningful life goals, reacts more slowly, is more self-accepting and less self-critical, and is more thoughtful, relaxed, and contemplative than the Type A counterpart. The Type B lifestyle is thought to be more conducive to health. Recent theories regarding A-B duality have been carefully scrutinized, especially in reference to increased health risk. Many of the original assumptions have not held true, but the high achiever with a stressful lifestyle often ignores bodily needs and is still thought to be at a higher risk for illness.

Some popular yet controversial current theories associate specific personality traits with certain illnesses. Recent literature has examined the question of a "cancer personality," the individual described as nice, accepting, polite, passive, sensitive, and subservient. Those with colon diseases are thought to be rigid, compulsive, and anxious. Those with rheumatoid arthritis are unable to express anger and are self-sacrificing, compliant, depressed, introverted and tense. Migraine sufferers are viewed as compulsive, perfectionistic, hostile, self-righteous, and rigid. Those prone to coronary disease are egotistical, unable to express resentment, and performance-oriented (Pelletier, 1977).

Such theories remain unproven. Whether certain personality traits precede an illness or develop as a result of the illness is also unknown. To associate an illness with a certain personality type is to run the risk of oversimplifying. However, it is highly possible that a busy, active type of person is predisposed to illness because of the high stress level in this type of lifestyle, and that in some people the immune system is inclined to be vulnerable for genetic or other reasons. On the other hand, Sara Reynolds, M.D., comments, "I know of no study of active overachievers with stress to see what proportion *don't* develop CFIDS."

PUTTING IT ALL TOGETHER

The microbe is nothing; the terrain everything.
J. Achterberg, *Imagery in Healing:*
Shamanism and Modern Medicine

We tend to oversimplify the problem, believing that a germ causes an illness; therefore, conquering the germ will allow us to become well again. The illness process is actually a complex interaction between a susceptible host and a triggering agent. The agent alone doesn't cause the illness; it acts as a catalyst in provoking the vulnerabilities of an organism.

The unicausal approach is tantalizingly simple. All we have to do is identify the culprit, kill that rotten germ, and be well again. But as in any war, the problem is not as simple as merely obliterating the enemy. That doesn't solve the problem; there will always be other enemies. Interaction between such factors as environment, heredity, behavior, infectious agents, immune functioning, central nervous system functioning, coping strategies, self-expectations, and stress are likely determinants of who will get ill and who will not. Other determinants of disease resistance include psychosocial factors such as lifestyle, job, place of residence, cultural background, personality factors, race, sex, and social status.

Causal hypotheses

Numerous hypotheses have been suggested about the cause of CFIDS. These are not mutually exclusive; many of them fit together nicely. Among them are the following:

- ✦ CFIDS is caused by a massive environmental assault (toxins, chemicals, stress, etc.), causing the immune system to succumb to major illness.

- ✦ A number of different causal agents produce the same basic type of syndrome in different people. Or two infectious agents hitting simultaneously may be necessary to produce the illness.

- ✦ Predisposing factors allow a single causal agent, which may be a virus, to cause infection in some of the people exposed to it. This infection causes disruption in the immune system (a failure to down-regulate, or chronic activation), causing susceptibility to a host of other infections.

✦ A causal agent causes the initial infection, disregulates the immune system, and allows previously dormant viruses (such as the herpesviruses) to come out of their latent state and begin to reproduce. The reaction of the immune system to this reactivation of viruses causes CFIDS symptoms.

✦ An already-damaged immune system is confronted with an assault by an agent but cannot properly handle the assault. As a result, various lymphokines (such as interleukin-2 and interferon) become elevated and cause CFIDS symptoms.

In his recent book *The Disease of a Thousand Names*, David Bell, M.D., presents variations on these themes, adding Variant Hypothyroidism Theory, Environmental Poison Theory, Abnormal Red Blood Cell Theory, Metabolic Myopathy Theory and Cytokine Theory. The cause is not likely to be explained by a single agent or in a simple way: CFIDS is a complex disease.

Jay Goldstein, M.D., views CFIDS as a multiphase illness. He writes a column explaining his theories in *The CFIDS Chronicle* and summarized his hypothesis about CFIDS at the October 1988 Rhode Island CFIDS Symposium. As the illness progresses from Phase I, in which agent *x* encounters immune cells, through additional phases in which the body reacts to the invader, immune functions become activated and body organs are affected. In the CFIDS patient, certain types of abnormal reactions create ongoing symptoms. He has described his proposed view of CFIDS as a five-phase process in his book, *CFS: The Struggle for Health*:

Phase Zero: Alteration of the immune system occurs, likely due to genetic predisposition.

Phase I: Viral infection occurs, with introduction of new viruses or reactivation of latent viruses.

Phase II: Immune disregulation develops. There is abnormal processing of antigens.

Phase III: Inappropriate types of cytokines are generated
in large numbers as disregulation of the immune
system continues.

Phase IV: Symptoms are manifested in different body
systems that have cytokine receptors, notably the
gastrointestinal tract and the central nervous system.

Phase V: Communication among immune system and
body organs is disrupted. Secondary illnesses develop.

A universal theme among CFIDS researchers is the emphasis
on immune disregulation. Jay Levy, M.D., has hypothesized that
AIDS research will be helpful to ongoing CFIDS research, that
the causative agent of CFIDS is most likely a common one
(that is, many people are infected but only some develop symptoms), that the agent may be difficult to spot because "it is kept
so far underground by the immunologic reaction" that it may
never be found, that CFIDS may be linked to multiple sclerosis
and other long-term illnesses, and that CFIDS is likely "an autoimmune reaction to *something*" (summary of the March 1989 San
Francisco CFS Conference, *The CFIDS Chronicle*, Spring 1989).

A second theme in current theory is involvement of the
central nervous system, especially the brain, as either the "site
of pathology" (Wakefield, November 1990, p. 45) or as the
system through which symptoms are transduced regardless of
the original cause of the illness (Goldstein, May 1991).
Goldstein views disregulation of the temporolimbic area of the
brain as central in producing CFIDS-associated symptoms and
proposes that CFIDS is a "limbic encephalopathy in a dysregulated neuroimmune network."

The lack of a unified hypothesis is due to several factors,
primarily ignorance—of the immune system, of the viral process, of the subtle interactions between and among body systems (notably the immune and nervous systems), and of the
interactions between organism and environment. We will need
to take a multifaceted approach to CFIDS in order to understand it. As research continues, we will no doubt uncover new
evidence regarding possible causative agents and contributory
factors.

PART II

CFIDS: What It Does

Chapter 8

◆

Effects of CFIDS
on Patients' Lives

Let me tell you that from a purely experiential, sensory perspective, CFIDS lives in the brain, and in the soul. It cripples the mind and the spirit as much as it does the body.

Marc Iverson
The CFIDS Chronicle

According to a recent poll of chronic Epstein-Barr [CFIDS] sufferers, 40 percent have been forced to leave their jobs or schooling. Marriages fall apart. Depression is a common complication. To these stresses add the unsympathetic skepticism of much of the medical community. "Massively overdiagnosed," "a vogue disease, like hypoglycemia," and "wastebasket diagnosis" are just some of the professional judgments that have found their way into print.

William Boly, "Raggedy Ann Town"

CFIDS SEEMS LIKE THE TYPE of incomprehensible thing that happens to other people. We become ill with a sense of disbelief and betrayal, as if we couldn't possibly be its targets. After all, we have an awful lot to do and don't have time for illness or limitations. And as the illness lingers it becomes more difficult to deny its foothold on our lives.

Just as a senseless death is a tragedy, so is a senseless life. As many PWCs have noted, AIDS kills you, whereas CFIDS kills your lifestyle, your hopes, and ambitions. Periodically you get some of it back, only to lose it again. The unpredictability of CFIDS presents a horrible challenge. The most severely affected people lead a day-to-day existence in which they are capable of taking care of only their most basic needs. Bedridden, they must depend on others financially and emotionally. In others the illness is cyclical: "down" periods are interspersed with more productive days.

Some PWCs describe the devastating effects of CFIDS:

With this illness, you don't have the concrete thing to look at, like a big lump on your arm. It's invisible. Not only is it invisible to everybody else, but you begin to think that maybe it really doesn't exist. I've tried to pretend that sometimes. My body had just crumbled. It was out of my control; that's the scary part. The ear thing, then the motion thing, then I couldn't drive anywhere, couldn't study, then I just couldn't function. Am I going to be incapacitated? Do I need a mental hospital? Am I dying? What is going on?

CFS has totally disrupted every aspect of my life!

It's been a two-and-a-half year nightmare experience.

This is a boring illness.

I feel like I've got permanent jet lag.

I used to watch kids in my home, but I kept falling asleep, and that's dangerous. I drank a lot of [caffeine] just to keep myself going through my routine without falling asleep. Sometimes my heart raced, or I got the shakes. I gained weight. I'd lose it, then get tired and gain it again. It seems to be a roller coaster; it never levels out. I can't control it. I'm used to controlling my life. Even when I do the things that I know are good for me, I expect that it will help, but sometimes nothing helps.

Life is passing me by.

I used to look forward to every day. Now I wake up and think "Oh shit, I'm awake." I wake up totally exhausted. I guess I only feel good when I'm sleeping.

My body is a traitor.

"[CFIDS] is capable of destroying the *experience* of life," wrote Hilary Johnson. "For me, CEBV [chronic Epstein-Barr Virus syndrome] has been the most wrenching, discouraging episode of my life, changing my relationship with the world. . . . [It is] a kind of endless mononucleosis with a touch of Alzheimer's disease." In Part II of her *Rolling Stone* article, she described fruitless attempts to maintain a positive attitude, but most often her mood was black and gloomy.

And everybody says, "I'm sick and tired of feeling sick and tired."

Many PWCs awaken feeling as tired as they did the night before, wondering, "How bad am I going to feel today?" We pay close attention to the nuances of our physical and emotional functioning, alert for the development of new symptoms, or old ones subsiding, or to a particularly "good" or "bad" day, seeking some sense of how well or poorly we will be able to function.

A good day (or week or hour) is to be treasured, its energy spent wisely, its pleasures fully savored. We are on leave from being sick but can be called back at any moment. We must be careful not to overdo, which will cut our good time short. We are ever alert for overt or subtle signs of a relapse.

On a bad day (or week or hour), time is interminable, life is bleak, and our goal is just to survive. Basic, routine activities, such as getting the mail and making minor decisions, turn into major tasks of enormous complexity. Kyle says, "I feel over-loaded, overwhelmed. There are many days when I feel like I can't handle one more thing. I've made so many major decisions in my life. Now 'What am I going to wear today?' is a major decision."

An excerpt from my journal reads:

On a good day I feel like I've got this thing licked for good. I know it can come back, but I figure I can roll with the cycle.

On a bad day I think I'll never in my whole life feel good again. I feel useless, worthless, drained, fat, and stupid. I hate being sick, and I hate myself, and I figure anyone who loves me is even crazier than I am.

It's impossible to prepare for continual readjustment. It's impossible to plan in advance or to make major commitments. Every tentative plan is carefully qualified with "maybe." My husband asks me if I'd like to go for a walk later, and I have no way of knowing if I'll be up to it.

Trying to make plans with someone who also has CFIDS is weird. "Would you like to come over on Saturday night about 8:00 if we're both feeling okay?" And the response: "Sure. I mean, maybe. I'll let you know on Saturday at 7:55."

When we feel sickest, we don't even care about getting together with friends or doing other things we used to enjoy. Lacking motivation and goals, we feel lazy and awful. We're too tired to *want to* want to do anything. "Deprivation of motivation is the greatest mental tragedy because it destroys all guidelines," wrote Hans Selye (1974).

What's left? Who cares? How long will I continue to feel this way? Forever? Pain, fear, and uncertainty. And then another breakthrough. Maybe this time it's really over. Maybe I'll just continue to improve from now on. It wasn't *that* bad feeling sick. And so it goes.

Uncertainty and unpredictability become the hallmarks of the new lifestyle, the one we grudgingly adopt. These themes permeate every aspect of our lives: self-image, self-esteem, career, finances, education, relationships, and recreation. Our roles in our families change, our feelings change, our bodies function strangely, doing unpredictable and uncomfortable things. Others don't understand. Friends, family, and doctors are puzzled by our altered behaviors and feelings. Our social roles change. We no longer contribute as we had and instead feel dependent and demanding. We lose a large degree of control over our lives. We have been sabotaged from within. Or from somewhere.

When questioned about the effects of CFIDS on their lives, PWCs in Phoenix, Arizona, responded:

	Positive Effect	Negative Effect
Employment	4%	91%
Relationship with significant other	18	70
Relationships with family	18	55
Relationships with friends	18	66
Financial status	2	74
Lifestyle in general	7	89
Personality in general	2	92

(The remainder experienced no effect)

Andy Rooney described having the flu as wanting only one thing: to recover. He noted how difficult it was to do such simple things as turn over and get up to go to the bathroom. "I'd lie in bed wondering how I'd feel if this were a disease I'd never get over" (1985, p. 197).

That's where we're stuck. This is like a flu that might get better, or better and then worse, or just stay the same. Everything we've ever planned is up for grabs.

ECONOMIC EFFECTS

Chronic illness creates financial dependency on others: spouse, parents, friends and families, and in some cases on private insurance and/or Social Security disability benefits. Because our abilities vary with the severity of the illness, dependency is a matter of degree. PWCs who filled out questionnaires and who discussed their situations with me expressed embarrassment, frustration, and helplessness because of their need to depend on others.

The results of a second questionnaire administered to Phoenix area PWCs indicated a dramatic change in work status since the onset of CFIDS.

	Pre-Illness	Since Illness
Work full-time	76%	11%
Work part-time	16	32
Not working	8	58

Another survey of 100 CFIDS patients indicated similar findings:

> ... [A]lthough 92% of the patients had been employed before they were diagnosed, only 65% were employed following onset of the illness. And, while 76% of the patients worked 40 or more hours per week before they became ill, 73% report working fewer than 40 hours after they became ill. (Staver, 1989)

A survey published in the Summer 1990 *Mass. CFIDS Update* indicated that 12% of PWCs worked full-time, 52% worked part-time, and 36% cannot work.

These figures show an especially marked shift in the numbers of people who worked full-time prior to the onset of CFIDS and who now work either part-time or not at all. The effects of CFIDS on patients' ability to participate productively in the work force have been drastic.

Men who are no longer able to work suffer the stigma of no longer being the breadwinner, wage earner, achiever—in short, an inability to fulfill the traditional male role. Women who fought the stereotype of the passive nonachieving female by becoming high achievers now find themselves disappointingly dependent on their spouses or families for support. PWCs in their late teens and early twenties, normally a time for establishing independence, find themselves thrust back into the role of dependent children. Giving up the roles and goals that helped to define us and give our lives meaning has been difficult. And on a more practical level, the financial crunch has ranged from difficult to devastating.

With her career plans interrupted indefinitely, Yolanda decided to apply for a low-stress job she felt she might be able to handle. Frustrated by her inability to continue with her original plans, she reluctantly lowered her sights.

> I'm not doing what I want to do, and I don't know how to accept that. I haven't given up on my career goals; I'm trying to be positive. I don't know whether to push myself or berate myself, to feel guilty because I couldn't cut it .... You need to

feel successful at something. I always wanted to do something other people saw as worthwhile to validate my self-worth. Out of guilt and self-incrimination, I've applied [for a menial job] for which I was overqualified. They asked why I wanted the job, and I couldn't just say "I have this virus." It was like, "I'm not the only one who wonders why I'm here." Other people wonder, too. I did a good rendition of "I've got to get on with my life."

Six months later Yolanda was relieved that she hadn't gotten the job because she wasn't sure she could handle its demands. Still, she felt that "If you're not earning a paycheck, you're not worth shit. My husband and even my children feel that way about it. I just feel useless." Her self-esteem had crumbled. Three years later Yolanda is divorced and remains unable to work.

Since so many of us had been strong, responsible people and since we still usually appear healthy, others' expectations of us remain constant. Our ability to achieve is severely impaired, however, and others are continually disappointed in our failure to function as we had previously.

Betty describes her difficult situation:

The head of the agency for which I worked really disappointed me. He kept saying, "You need to rest and take care of yourself because we need you. You've always produced for us." I thought, "You son of a gun," but I just said, "I can't right now. I can't concentrate. I can't absorb what I read." [He demanded] a lot of me, researching and drafting important information. He said, "It's just a virus, so just work for a couple of hours and go home and rest and you'll do all right. You come back in the morning, and the work will just come pouring out. Don't do anything at home. Rest at home; don't cook, don't do the laundry." He was making more and more demands. One of my close friends said, "Tell him to go fuck himself. Why are you letting him do this?" I said, "I cannot let him down. I can't let my family down. I can't let anybody down."

But she was letting all of them down, and by disappointing others she was also letting herself down. Quitting her job and learning to relax was a difficult but eye-opening experience for Betty, who found that her department did continue to function in her absence. She learned to take it easy and to enjoy her life more fully. Six months later, Betty reported a considerable degree of recovery, but she wasn't nearly ready to return to work. The good news: she no longer felt responsible or guilty for her inability to work as she had before.

Kyle describes a different predicament: previously an energetic worker, and now with limited energy and poor health, she was about to separate from her husband.

> Now I'm getting ready to live on my own, and I don't think I can do that because of the disease. I'm just not strong enough to make it on my own because I just can't think the way I used to or do the things I used to do. What if I have a relapse and can't work? What am I going to do?

Other PWCs comment:

> I was at the height of my career when this thing struck. [This statement has been made by countless PWCs.]

> I'm the kind of guy who never falls apart. I'm always fair and honest and was always a good problem solver and a hard worker. I can't do that now; I can't do the kind of job I can feel good about, so I don't work at all. It's a big hurdle for a Type A, workaholic, hard-driving, very successful, polyphasic thinker who loves what he does to change the rules. These are abrupt changes, and you can't make them . . . very easily. Nothing like this has ever happened to me before.

> My worst fear is being dependent.

> My security got taken away.

> I'm terrified that it will never go away and I will lie in bed the rest of my life with only the TV, magazines and pets. There is no joy or fun in my life; I'm a burden. I can't participate in work or community activities. I can't get out of bed.

> I no longer feel productive. What's left?

My life has become centered only in work because that's all I have energy to do.

I will have to retire earlier than I had planned.

These people have expressed some of the common reactions among those of us who can no longer function as we used to and whose careers, educational plans, and incomes have been drastically affected by CFIDS.

Although many have stopped working, some have continued to work either because their illness is less severe or because they feel they must continue for financial reasons or a personal need not to "give in" to the illness. The work ethic is thoroughly instilled in us; not to work is not okay. Those who push on despite a significant degree of illness admit that they may be jeopardizing their health and prolonging the illness but feel that leaving work is simply not an option. Their self-expectations remain constant and high. However, some are later forced to quit when they can no longer function in the workplace. It is a source of shame not to be able to carry on despite the illness, to be unable to prove that we can overcome this obstacle.

Whether to continue with work and/or school, and to what degree, becomes a matter of individual judgment. It makes sense to continue meaningful activities to the extent possible but not to the point at which chances of recovery are jeopardized. The advice to continue with what you are doing to whatever degree is comfortable for you at a given time requires difficult evaluations, flexibility, common sense, and guesswork. It means being honest with yourself about what is feasible, shedding unrealistically heroic self-expectations. Inability to work usually causes loss of benefits coupled with soaring medical expenses. Even when an individual has health insurance, many treatments are not covered. Some policies contain a catch-22 clause stating that only standard treatment for an illness is covered, and there is no standard treatment for CFIDS at this time. Many PWCs have exhausted their incomes and even savings accounts seeking helpful treatment.

Self-esteem plummets along with income, and the loss of one's identity as a productive worker is significant. One option for those who can no longer work is to apply for disability benefits. However, the application process is often long and frustrating, and the notion of relying on insurance companies and on the government for support is difficult to accept for those who are career-oriented. Social Security Disability Income (SSDI) benefits have been difficult to obtain for many PWCs. The Social Security manual lists an illness called "Chronic Epstein-Barr Virus Syndrome," stating that onset, duration, severity, and residual ability to function are factors to be considered in determining if benefits are to be awarded. Obtaining these benefits is not automatic for "CEBV" patients. Because the "CEBV" diagnosis is inaccurate and inappropriate, many PWCs have applied for benefits on the basis of multisystem impairments or mood disorders. Most commonly SSDI applications are turned down because of a lack of understanding of CFIDS by Social Security personnel, although the Social Security Administration indicates that administrative law judges are being educated about CFIDS. PWCs are often denied benefits in the first two stages of applying for benefits, which are handled at the state level. This decision can and should be appealed but the process is long, arduous, and frustrating. Ultimately, many PWCs are able to obtain benefits but there is a long time lapse between the initial application and the final decision. Similar problems may be encountered with private disability insurance claims.

CFIDS can devastate one's lifestyle, bank balance, career, and educational plans. Illness can force us to incur large debts (because of decreased income and increased medical expenses) or to move to less expensive housing or "back home." Most PWCs have experienced a decrease in their standard of living, and many find their financial futures disturbingly uncertain.

EFFECTS OF CFIDS ON SELF-IMAGE

Self-image is the way we view ourselves. Self-esteem is how we feel about ourselves, our sense of personal value and worth. CFIDS affects both dramatically. "Before I got sick," says Lorna . . .

I was vivacious, outgoing, always "up." I was the achiever, the giver, the caretaker. I was a successful salesperson. I felt I could do anything I wanted to do. Now I have mood fluctuations, I become depressed, and even have thoughts of committing suicide. I'm vulnerable; I've lost my identity and my self-esteem. I can't work, and I can't even be a good mother to my two-year-old son. I feel guilty because I have nothing to give to others. We're having financial problems because I can no longer work. I can't concentrate, I have blackouts, I lose my train of thought. I'm weak and numb much of the time.

Suddenly everything is different; we are unaccustomed to the new, unwelcome feelings and perceptions. We must redefine ourselves and our lives. I wrote in my journal about my lost sense of self. I felt like a victim of bizarre internal circumstances beyond my control, having become in essence a stranger to myself.

Paula says:

My self-esteem went right down because I couldn't do things. It wasn't that I didn't want to. I did want to, but I couldn't. I'd never been helpless in my life; I've always been fiercely independent, radically so. I never needed any help. So when I started having to ask, I didn't ask. I kept struggling to try to do and got angry at the people around me. And their expectations of me, because this is what I'd trained them to expect, was that I could do it . . . better than anyone. All of a sudden, I couldn't. This was my whole lifestyle, my mindset, my whole core of who I am . . . and now I'm not who I was. I can't do it.

Are we victims? We feel a loss of control regarding our plans for the present and the future. Helplessness feels alien, uncomfortable, and dangerous. Martin Seligman (1975) has written about the loss of control that accompanies certain life events, pointing out the correlations between helplessness and depression. When we lack control and predictability in our lives, we begin to feel hopeless, helpless, and weak.

The onset and continuation of CFIDS provokes such feelings, which exert a negative influence on the illness process, compounding the problems and crushing our self-perceptions, self-expectations, and hopes. In the words of PWCs:

> I am so much less myself.

> I want to be productive. I used to think I could be perfect if I tried hard enough.

> I was this superperson. Under stress, I just pushed harder. It worked for all those years.

> I feel so stupid now. My brain doesn't work. I can't even do simple things, like type.

> I was taught to be strong. Now I don't have the strength to get up off the floor. I feel I have failed my family, my co-workers, myself.

> The uncertainty is awful. Will I be an invalid for the rest of my life? [Feeling like an "invalid" means feeling "in-valid."]

> My sense of humor . . . I don't think I've lost it, but I have to fake it; life has become a lot more serious. I'm overly sensitive now. And when someone's fuckin' with me, I don't understand what they're doing, and I take it seriously, whereas before I used to know and laugh. I'm not as bizarre as I used to be; I've really toned down. I can't joke because my brain can't come up with anything smart. I'm too serious.

> The worst thing that could happen has happened. My mind's functioning has been impaired. I can handle pain or other kinds of physical discomfort. This affects me, myself; it's the hardest thing to handle. The uncertainty of not knowing if I'm going to be me again.

> I used to be successful, aggressive, fast-moving, and I thrived on it. My profession was lucrative. But I can't function like that any more. I can hardly function at all, period. I do the best I can, but I'm not the same guy I used to be.

> I don't know what I'm capable of doing. I wish someone could tell me what to do and what not to do. Then I wouldn't feel guilty about all the things I'm not doing.

> My psychiatrist told me I may never be well enough to [resume former activities]. I have trouble with "never" and "may never," with not knowing.

> I was trained to be "fine." You're supposed to always be fine.

We define ourselves largely in terms of what we do. Indeed, this is usually the first question new acquaintances will ask each other. In college it was "What's your major?" and later it was "What do you do?" How do we answer that question when we can no longer function in accustomed roles? Options: *I sleep. I stay in bed a lot. I do what I can. I work part-time. I collect disability payments. I complain a lot.* These are all true, but not happily so. Who am I without my former roles? We have become human doings rather than human beings, as John Bradshaw said in his PBS lecture series.

Everything we knew about ourselves before is now up for grabs. We apply new labels to ourselves, many of them hurtful and self-deprecating. *Am I a hypochondriac?* (I'm certainly obsessed with my body and its functioning.) *Am I a dependent person?* (I have far greater needs than in the past.) *Am I a sickie?* (This illness dominates my life to an uncomfortably great degree.) *Am I a patient?* (I hate that passive-sounding word, and I'm not at all patient about this illness.) *Am I a pessimist? Or a realist?* (It's hard to be hopeful sometimes, especially when symptoms hit unpredictably.) *Am I a survivor?* (Or does that mean I'm pushing too hard and risking self-harm?) *Am I a martyr?* (That's how I feel when I perform resentfully, out of a sense of duty, even though I'm too drained to function well.) *Am I a grouch?* (I get angry over nothing, and I'm very angry about being ill.)

Like the labels, our self-messages are often negative and irrational, reflecting changes in self-image and self-esteem. Examples of damaging, often irrational self-messages are:

> I can't do anything any more.

> I'll always be this way; I'll never get better.

> I brought this on myself. It's my fault that I'm sick.

If I could think positively, I could banish this illness.

I should fake it, play the "I'm fine" game. I'm acceptable to myself and others only when I'm well.

I need to be taken care of, and that's a sign of weakness.

I shouldn't complain.

I used to be superwoman/superman, superemployee, super-friend, superparent. Now I'm superwimp.

I shouldn't be so down, so depressed.

I should be able to change this, make it go away.

I'm supposed to be strong, capable of anything, able to handle the responsibilities of the world.

I'm too sensitive. I shouldn't feel or react as I do.

I used to think I was smart, but now I know I'm stupid.

My life is over.

Such distorted, unrealistic, perfectionistic self-statements compound the already numerous problems of chronic illness.

Kyle summarizes her situation well:

I'm not the same person. I can't think and speak like I could before. I can't make the decisions I used to make. I'm different than other people, and people don't understand what's going on with me. I want to say, "Hey, I'm not really stupid. I have this virus." I want to wear it on a badge: *Please don't think I'm an idiot.*

I had a real full life, and I don't any more. My brain isn't the same anymore. Things are fragmented, and sometimes I even have trouble talking, putting sentences together. I'll be in the middle of the most profound thing in the world, and I'll forget what I was saying.

I feel really ripped off. I can't lead a normal life. I don't have a whole lot of energy. I don't have a normal social life. I have to go to bed at nine o'clock. I live a pretty one-dimensional life where I go to work and come home and spend the evening in my recliner . . . .

I feel like my brain will never be the same and I'll never be the same person I was before, even if I recover.

But look how much we can cope with. We've been to hell and back, and back and forth again, and we've made it through. We are survivors, and we deserve full credit for our endurance.

FEELINGS

Feelings are pure emotion, irrational by definition. We can't talk ourselves out of them, but we need to define and understand them and their effects. It's also helpful to know how others in similar circumstances feel, so we don't feel so alone and crazy.

The gamut of CFIDS-triggered emotions include feeling:

Guilty. Did I cause my illness? Did I choose to become ill? Is this "mind over matter"? Am I being punished for a wrongdoing? Am I somehow keeping myself from getting well? Is there something else I should be doing, or something I'm not doing right? I can't work any longer, or I don't work as productively as I should. I'm spending too much money on treatments that might not even work. I shouldn't have so many special needs. I'm letting everyone down, disappointing them—family, friends, employer, and myself. Maybe those who think I'm not really sick are right after all, and I'm just copping out. I don't have fewer responsibilities when I'm sick, just extra guilt for not carrying them out.

Misunderstood. No one else really understands what I'm going through, except (maybe) the others who have it, too. Those close to me may try to understand, and think they understand, but they really can't. If I didn't have CFIDS, I wouldn't be able to understand what it's like, either, I suppose. I feel isolated and rejected.

Overloaded. Even simple tasks overwhelm me. I can't make decisions. I can't sort things out. I can't trust myself to judge the degree of a problem or to know how to react in proportion to its significance. Molehills become mountains, and I don't always know when I'm distorting.

Depressed. Sometimes things are so bleak, disappointing, and pointless. I feel incapable and unlovable. Sometimes I cry over nothing; other times I need to cry but can't. There's nothing I value or enjoy. Life is just one empty moment after another, interminably. Everything takes too much effort; nothing is worth doing. I'm not spontaneous or creative or fun-loving or silly any more. I'm a blob.

Desperate. There's no hope. I've tried various remedies and interventions, even weird stuff, and nothing has worked well enough. Maybe nothing ever will. If only I knew what to do, I'd do it—whatever it was.

Suicidal. Why don't I just die now? There's nothing left; my life is the pits. If I can't lead a useful life, I might as well not exist. I'd rather die than continue to exist like this. I need to get well or to die.

Marc Iverson, president of The CFIDS Association of Charlotte, North Carolina, says:

> I have never known a person with full-blown CFIDS who has not considered suicide at some point in his or her illness. I have known a number of individuals with this disease who have chosen death . . . . CFIDS steals so much of their lives that life is simply not worth living. (November 1990)

Isolated. Sometimes I don't want to be alone, but I don't want to be with anyone either. Others can't possibly understand my feelings; I have no way of explaining them. Come closer; go away. Accompanied or alone, I live in a private hell. There's an invisible wall between me and the rest of the world.

Crazy. Is this real? Have I lost my mind? CFIDS is a hall of mirrors from hell, distorted and freaky. I was level-headed and able to cope, but I've gone off the deep end. I don't even know who I am. Awake and asleep, my thoughts are distorted. I don't understand my thoughts, my feelings, or myself. I'm not normal now, not myself anymore.

Sad. I've lost so much. This is so difficult. I've been taught to look on the bright side, but right now there isn't one. Everything hurts—my body, but also my heart, my spirit.

Stunned. I can't believe this is happening to me. I cannot accept this illness.

Deprived. There are so many things I can't do and things I shouldn't do or eat or drink. What's left? I want a normal life back. My life has been pulled out from under me; so much has been torn away.

Uncertain. Will this ever be over? Will I ever feel good again? When? How will I feel tomorrow? How will I feel in an hour? Why did this happen? Do I dare make any plans? Do I dare to have hopes and dreams?

Confused. I don't understand what's happening to me. I can't make sense out of this predicament; I just know it feels bad. I can't trust myself to think or react rationally and logically.

Helpless. I feel like an out-of-control victim, an unacceptable role for me. I'm so vulnerable physically and emotionally. My whole life is now unpredictable. I'm being held hostage by something mysterious and elusive. No one even knows what this illness really is. You can't *see* an immune system or know what's going wrong. There's not a damned thing I can do about it, either. I'm trapped inside a body that doesn't work right and won't cooperate. I don't have any faith in my abilities, my competence. I don't have the resources to fix this or even to adapt. The rules keep changing and all I can do is react.

Dependent. I'm useless, worthless. I am forced to rely upon others to do the things I should be able to do and used to do. It's hard to feel good about me or to view myself as capable when I'm so dependent on others. I used to be in the driver's seat; now I'm just a passenger. I used to be a giver; now I'm a taker. It's not okay to be so needy.

Self-absorbed. I get so wrapped up in how I'm feeling that I lose awareness of how others feel or what they need. Or if I am aware, sometimes I don't even have the energy to care. That's not like me. All I think about is this illness and what it's doing to me. My entire focus is inward; I'm preoccupied with my symptoms, worrying and wondering what they mean and what lies ahead for me.

Debilitated. I have no energy. I feel used up. The vital part of me is gone.

Angry. Why do bad things happen to good people? Why me? I hate this; it's unfair. Why can't someone fix me, make me better? I've tried so hard, and I've done so well; why am I being punished? This illness doesn't follow the rules. I *hate* CFIDS.

Weak. I can't take care of myself or my own life. I'm a wimp now. My body is weak; my mind doesn't work right. I'm inadequate, wimpy.

Afraid. What will happen to me? Will I become sicker? Will I develop new, worse symptoms? Lose even more control? Will I get cancer? Die? My head is filled with frightening possibilities, and no one has answers; nobody can assure me the worst won't happen. I'm afraid I'll never get well. I'm afraid of what I can't identify and don't understand.

Numb. I feel dull, flat. This may be a temporary escape from emotional pain, but I can't feel pleasure either. I feel nothing.

Resigned. It will always be like this. It's endless. They'll never find a cure, or even a remedy. It's hopeless; I might as well get used to it. My life as I knew it is over.

Hopeful. Maybe there will be a breakthrough. Some people recover; maybe I'll be one of them. I just have to get better; I have to believe I will. Someday I'll look back on all of this . . .

Relieved. It is possible to feel good, even if only for brief periods of time. I haven't forgotten how. There's hope.

The feelings vacillate unpredictably and uncomfortably, often triggered by a symptom exacerbation. All these feelings are natural reactions to an unpredictable, chronic illness. We must learn to recognize and express these feelings despite their seeming irrationality. There are no shortcuts, and feelings don't go away if they're ignored; they go underground. Unexpressed emotions fester and will ultimately spill out inappropriately, causing damage to relationships. Repressed feelings may further compromise the immune system.

EFFECTS OF CFIDS ON RELATIONSHIPS

Today, who needs a physician
When every friend is a diagnostician?
Ogden Nash, "We're Fine, Just Fine"

Attitudes and beliefs of others about CFIDS

With the onset of CFIDS, others in our lives are puzzled but often sympathetic. As time goes on, they may begin to doubt the existence of an invisible malady, wondering if the illness is real. The PWC may feel betrayed while experiencing self-doubt as well, compounding an already painful situation.

Once we obtain a diagnosis of "chronic fatigue syndrome" it's hard to get others to take it seriously. It sounds too much like "chronic complainer's syndrome" or "crazy and lazy disease." We finally get a name for it, but by then everyone's run out of patience, and the name itself doesn't add much credibility. Calling it CFIDS may help the credibility factor somewhat.

There are two aspects of chronic illness: the obvious, physiological, tangible signs, and the hidden difficulties. The obvious signs identify one as sick and are usually taken seriously. The hidden ones are made evident to others only by verbal reports. If there is a discrepancy between the two (no obvious symptoms but reports of feeling awful), others become confused and have a hard time grasping the true nature and severity of the illness. Our society looks for evidence; seeing is believing. If you can't see it, it's not there. The assumption is that the severity of one's illness is directly proportional to its degree of visibility.

During the years that I have had CFIDS I've looked okay most of the time. Those closest to me have learned to read my signals of impending fatigue, often before I'm aware of them. They notice paleness, a general slowing down, and/or increased sensitivity to sensory input. However, to the casual observer I appear fine. No problem. I even feel strange telling others how lousy I feel, so I don't unless there's a good reason. I know it's hard for them to understand what they cannot see and have not experienced. The most distressing aspects of CFIDS are invisible. With no bandages, casts, spots, bruises, or other obvious signs of illness, I am presumed well.

Since we may look fine while feeling horrible, others' expectations of us remain about the same. And often others may harbor erroneous assumptions about CFIDS:

If it's not terminal, it's no big deal. Others sometimes think we should just get on with our lives as before and stop paying attention to symptoms, stop worrying, and stop pampering ourselves (e.g., resting so much). Yolanda says, "When I first got sick, everyone was concerned, but now it's last year's news. People feel like if it's not fatal, it should be gone by now." They run out of patience, just as we do.

It's a woman's disease. Although a greater proportion of PWCs are female, women have not cornered the market on this disease. To call it a women's disease is not only to misrepresent the patient population but also to define the illness as a sex-linked affliction of an hysterical, not-quite-together, hormone-driven population.

It's an emotional disorder. The theory that this illness is merely depression with a dash of anxiety is unfair and perjorative. It ignores a whole host of CFIDS symptoms that have never been linked to depression. Such comments as "You're probably over-stressed," "You're just depressed and/or anxious," "You're just not handling stress very well," or "It's an attitude problem" add insult to illness.

It's related to AIDS. There is no known connection between CFIDS and HIV. Some patients report that others are afraid to be near them for fear of catching the illness. The stigma can result in needless fear and isolation. The unfortunate phobic response of many people to AIDS is thus transferred to CFIDS.

It must be curable. There must be something you can do to function normally. You get sick, you take medicine, you get better, right? Doing the right thing should restore health. We obviously lack the proper resources—willpower, determination, the right diet, medicine or exercise program.

If you complain, you're being negative. If you don't complain, you must be feeling okay. This is a double bind for the PWC, who must decide whether to fake it, ignore it, or describe the feelings and symptoms honestly. We're almost always aware of our symptoms and the reactions of others. We want our "invisible" illness to be acknowledged but sometimes it's simpler to play the game of ignoring it, which seems the acceptable thing to do. But when we put on an "I'm fine" act, others are fooled into believing that we are.

Our attempts to disguise or minimize our illness may backfire. Well-intentioned others often make insensitive comments such as:

> You're sick? You look fine to me!
>
> Maybe this illness is all in your imagination.
>
> Do you *still* have that illness?
>
> I've heard that CFIDS/CFS/CEBV doesn't really exist.
>
> There must be *something* you haven't tried that would cure you.
>
> You're lucky to rest and sleep all the time and stay home from work.
>
> Cheer up. Things could be worse.
>
> Your symptoms are the same ones everyone has.
>
> Maybe you just need more exercise or vitamins.

You just don't *want* to do stuff any more.

I think you just enjoy being sick—especially all the attention you get.

I know just how you feel.

Here's the one no one says, but it comes through loud and clear: *You're not allowed to be sick.*

People react in a variety of ways to chronic illness, depending upon their own psychological makeup and issues, their perceptions of illness, and their belief systems. Our society encourages denial of all things unpleasant, especially those we fear and/or cannot readily understand. A lingering and debilitating yet invisible illness can be a trigger for such a need to avoid and distance. Our pain and helplessness—and the fact that it could happen to them—makes others back away, and we attribute such behavior to lack of caring. Others' reactions have more to do with them than with us, but it's difficult to see this when we're vulnerable.

Effects of CFIDS on relationships with spouses/partners

"In sickness and in health" takes on a whole new meaning. We repeat that phrase automatically when we marry but have little insight into its implications. Initially, a shared tragedy may bring partners closer together, but as time goes on and the problem endures, the marriage may not. The divorce rate for couples in which one partner has a chronic illness is estimated at 75% (Pitzele, 1986, p. 64).

The PWC is needy, requiring attention, costly medical services, and financial and emotional support. The PWC is demanding, but not purposely so, usually feeling guilty for being burdensome, for not contributing as in the past, and for having so many needs. If the PWC had once been the primary caregiver in a relationship and can no longer fulfill this role, a significant adjustment must take place for the relationship to survive.

Caregivers have special needs, too, which may remain dangerously unexpressed because, after all, they are well and may feel guilty about having needs. Thus, the needs of the healthy partner may be overlooked. Maggie Strong writes in *Mainstay* about the greater burden on the well partner, who must assume an increased workload while the ill partner occupies center stage with his or her additional needs.

The major financial burden often falls upon the well partner. Sacrifices become necessary. Life with a sick person becomes monotonous and boring. Plans must be canceled, dreams and ambitions put on hold. Many major decisions are dictated by CFIDS, but the caregiver is expected to remain understanding and patient. One partner said, "It's awful being around a person who's always depressed and lethargic. She doesn't accomplish anything; she feels lousy all the time," adding that he really wanted to be understanding but just couldn't understand what she was experiencing or why she was so needy and so unlike her "past self."

Several spouses of PWCs complain about the dual financial burdens of decreased income compounded by high medical bills. While indicating a desire to help, they also distrust many health practitioners and costly treatment programs. The burden of providing financially means spending money on what some refer to as "quack remedies" that are expensive and of questionable value. The unspoken attitude seems to be, "With me spending all this money, the least she or he could do is get well," an understandable but unreasonable position. While some feel ripped off, others are determined to pursue treatment regardless of cost. All seem to be fed up with the illness that has destroyed their family's financial stability and, in some cases, their self-image as good providers.

Problems that existed in relationships prior to the onset of CFIDS will be compounded by it. Changes occur in role expectations—the part each spouse is expected to play—and couples do not make this transition easily. Too often the issues aren't even discussed. To push on grimly and silently is considered the heroic course, yet the unexpressed but mounting feelings of pressure and resentment damage the relationship.

Although stereotypical male and female roles are currently undergoing change, men have typically been regarded as the primary wage earners and women as the emotional caretakers in the family. When the husband is ill, the wife continues her caretaker role and may need to become the sole breadwinner as well. When the wife becomes ill, the husband is forced into a new role of emotional caretaker as well as financial provider. The financially and emotionally dependent spouse is prone to substantial guilt feelings.

If the ill spouse is a hard-driving female "achiever," illness may thrust her back into a dependent relationship with which she is uncomfortable. Having developed career and educational goals, and having obtained satisfaction, competence, self-esteem, and independence, she is once again thrust into a role from which she has been trying to escape: the dependent wife.

Many PWCs have been problem solvers, fixers, doers, and caretakers, often taking responsibility for finding solutions to others' problems. This codependency creates a bind when their own CFIDS-generated problems are not readily "fixable."

A partner who is a "fixer" may offer suggestions and advice. If the ill spouse does not follow the advice, the "fixer" may become angry at this lack of cooperation. If the ill spouse complies but the remedy is unsuccessful, the "fixer" may feel the need to blame either the ill spouse or him/herself for this failure. Rather than letting this dysfunctional blaming situation develop, it is far wiser to examine one's self-expectations regarding problem solving. Some problems are just not easily fixed, even when motivation to pursue solutions is strong. Often, the fixer is unaware that what the partner needs is support and understanding rather than well-intended but often ineffectual advice.

Illness (or any other continuing problem) can become the primary focus of a relationship. Like work, the role of illness expands to fit the time (and attention) available. A great deal of a couple's attention can be focused on CFIDS but a functional relationship requires that priorities be balanced.

When asked about the frequency of sexual activity prior to and after the onset of CFIDS, 79% of the respondents in a Phoenix survey indicated that sexual activity was less frequent, and only 18% said sexual frequency was about the same. (One person indicated that sex was more frequent, and she wrote an explanation in the margin: "Just married!") Many PWCs report that their sex drive has diminished substantially; others indicate that they just don't have the energy to have sex. A few reported that they enjoyed sex because it provided a brief "escape" from illness, a time when they could forget, but others said that sexual exertion caused a mild relapse over the next few days, so they were forced to weigh desire against consequences. What a shame to waste all that time spent in bed!

There's also the "come close, go away" syndrome, in which the PWC needs to be touched and comforted and simultaneously wants to crawl into a black hole of isolation. This sends out a confusing double message that may cause the partner to feel rejected.

Many PWCs are afraid. What if my illness and I are successful at pushing my partner away? What if my mate becomes fed up with the "sickie" I've become and leaves me? Yolanda is afraid her husband will leave her, and that she will be both emotionally bereft and financially destitute, since she can no longer work.

> A few weeks ago, it blew up, and he said he just couldn't handle being around a sick person. I've tried very hard not to act like a sick person; I don't stay in bed; I try to do the household work. But I have so much guilt and feelings of worthlessness because I've been so goal-oriented all my life, and now I'm so insecure. He usually blows up periodically and then it will pass over, but I'm afraid one of these times, he'll just leave.

In some cases spouses ultimately learn how to understand and handle the stressors presented by illness and grow closer. But in the face of pre-existing relationship problems compounded by the effects of a chronic illness, many relationships do not survive when the need to distance increases and understanding runs thin.

At times the need to communicate is strong, but the words won't come. This is in part the result of an inability to express these new feelings, compounded by CFIDS-related cognitive difficulties: impaired concentration, memory, and word-finding abilities. "I know what I want to say to [my partner]," says Kyle, "but I get confused and screw it up, and it starts a fight." She has trouble getting to the point because she loses it. The words become jumbled. The message becomes distorted or is incomplete, and both parties end up frustrated.

The PWC who had been an active and contributing partner is now depleted, robbing the healthy spouse of a challenging companion. Communication becomes strained and difficult as cognitive dysfunction increases. The well partner may retreat from the PWC, whose conversation has begun to focus on symptoms, losses, and other trials of CFIDS. The result is loss and loneliness for both partners.

But many are weathering the storm well. Many PWCs have expressed appreciation of understanding, supportive partners. Many partners express considerable caring, as well as the pain of being unable to make it okay for their loved ones. PWCs often refer to their partners as the strongest sources of support available, willing to listen, empathize, and problem-solve. Many caregivers read CFIDS literature and attend support group meetings with their ill partners. This willingness to learn, understand, and participate facilitates a couple's adjustment to CFIDS. One PWC reported:

> My husband knows that I can't do things even if I try. He has come to accept it and has become stronger as I've become weaker. It's been good for him, although it's been hard for both of us.

My husband has been my primary source of support. He's tolerated my mood swings: often I have snapped at him about the dumbest things and later he will say, "I guess that was CFIDS talking." His understanding and tolerance make me feel valued and cherished, but also guilty. Would I be able to do the same for him? CFIDS has spoiled so many of our plans; I've become a stick-in-the-mud. In some ways he's been ripped off as much as I have. But he sticks around, and we fight it to-gether. His caring overwhelms me at times. When I'm in an exacerbation accompanied by one of those life-shattering depressions, I don't understand how anyone could love me—but somehow he does. We still have good moments to share, in fact more and more frequently, and I am so grateful for the good times.

"My wife has been great," says Bill. "I'd like to think I'd be as good to her as she has been to me, but I don't know. What I've put her through is a very good test of [whether] she loves me."

But the illness remains a lurking enemy in our households, producing tension and disruption. Even with the knowledge that the problem is the illness rather than a lack of love between partners, old problems escalate and new ones develop. It's tough to hang together and work as a partnership with CFIDS in the way.

Effects of CFIDS on families

Some of the changes produced by chronic illness are PWCs' inability to shoulder former responsibilities, changes in financial circumstances, a shift in family priorities, new needs, and the feelings of confusion, anger, and resentment that develop. The PWC may feel guilty for causing problems and being a burden. Healthy family members may feel guilty because they were spared and resentful that the patient was not. In addition, the family accompanies the patient on the exacerbation-remission roller coaster; family life becomes more unpredictable. The PWC's anger may become disruptive since we often vent anger inappropriately at those we love and spend the most time with. Even when we understand what's happening and why, we must deal with changes: new roles, needs, demands, feelings, and losses —of predictability, of the PWC as we knew him or her before, of what was normal. Family members often feel guilty about expressing their own feelings and needs, trying to protect the sick person from feeling responsible for the changes and difficulties.

The family experiences a difficult period of adjustment in attempts to restore homeostasis, a sense of balance. This process is different for everyone, but it follows closely the pattern experienced in grieving. The family's ability to cope depends on its resources and pre-illness level of functioning. Adjustment requires flexibility, tolerance of change, and ability to acknowledge and communicate about what is happening. Family members are called upon to accommodate new needs and limitations of the PWC and to accept new responsibilities and roles. Together and individually they experience pain and disappointment. They must learn to do what is helpful for the ill family member without going to either extreme: denying the problem or becoming overprotective.

Family disruptions may impact the patient by causing an exacerbation of symptoms, which further stresses the family. "They were used to me always being in charge of everything," says Betty. "I went from supermom to superwimp." The transition is hard on everyone in the family.

My children have experienced difficulty with several aspects of my illness: my tendency to overreact or to react unpredictably, limitations on activities and travel plans, and changes in financial circumstances. Not only was I financially unable to provide for myself and my children as before, but a messy battle with my exhusband for increased child support ensued and the kids and my current spouse got caught up in the turmoil. Talking helps, but the problems continue.

One patient's small son said, "When are we going to get Mommy back?" Their mother used to take the kids to the park daily despite a hectic work schedule; she laughed and played with them a lot. Now she cries often, and her husband has assumed many of her former responsibilities. She says her whole family felt robbed.

Bill found himself overreacting to the behavior of his three young children because of CFIDS-related mood swings:

> I haven't been a good dad; I haven't been able to discipline my kids appropriately. I haven't been able to spend the time I normally would have spent with the kids, and that's killing me. It's one of the saddest things I've ever experienced; it's the hardest thing I've ever handled . . . . Before I was sick, I was able to get out with my oldest and do some things I haven't

been able to do with the others. They're always energetic, jumping around; they always want to be doing stuff. I can't do it. I do push myself; I go out with them even if I feel crummy. I want them to have a good experience. I don't know how my wife can handle all this; she has a real even temper.

Feelings of denial, guilt, anger, jealousy and depression are normal reactions of children to a parent's illness. Open discussion is helpful in allowing children to express these feelings and have them validated. Professional intervention may be required if their reactions are prolonged or particularly severe or if other danger signals are present, including rebelliousness, problems with schoolwork, substance abuse, and signs of depression.

We may resent the needs of our children at times, but it's a displaced resentment. What we really resent is our illness preventing us from parenting as we'd like to. We worry that our children will be deprived of what they deserve and would have had if we weren't ill. Will they look back on their childhoods and feel resentment? Probably—but all children feel resentful and must learn that many of their expectations will not be met. We can easily become overly concerned with pleasing our children. Unfortunately, they're subject to the same disappointments as the rest of us. We can't shield them, nor should we. They, too, must learn to cope.

Relationships with our extended families are likely to change. As we become adults, we perceive our parents as peers (with some parental undertones). When CFIDS intervenes, the roles change. Parents fall into their former parental roles again with the concomitant worry, need to give advice, and feelings of responsibility. They still want to make it all better and may try to deny the illness because of their own feelings of helplessness.

A curious role reversal takes place. Parents, even retired ones, may be leading active lives despite the inevitable aches and pains that accompany advancing age, while their children with CFIDS experience memory loss, arthritic-type pain, a sedentary lifestyle, and other symptoms and deficits that, in the scheme of things, are supposed to happen first to older people. The process reverses itself; I *feel* older than my parents *are*. I have many of the same problems with my illness that they have with advancing age. We may feel ashamed to rely on our parents again: "Here I am again, needing more parenting—emotionally and financially." It's a lousy feeling. It interrupts the natural life cycle by making us feel like dependent middle-aged children.

As Paula's mother has gotten older, she has increasingly relied on Paula for emotional support. Paula's role has been that of the giver, the caretaker, the listener—and now she has CFIDS.

> It's been hard for me to say "I need." I've never said that. I'm still in a supportive role with my mother and grandmother. My mother is just beginning to understand that I can no longer do many things. I always tried to live up to her expectations, but now she has to understand that there's something going on that I have no control over. Prior to that, her attitude was, "I know you're sick, but you're still functioning," along with her usual expectations. Now it's "Are you up to it? Do you feel like you can make it?"—not a demand, but a request. In this way, my relationships with people have gotten better.

In all family relationships, illness presents a challenge. It shakes up the status quo and demands new changes. Families who are able to work together, drawing on collective resources to meet the new challenges, become stronger as a result.

Effects of CFIDS on friendships

CFIDS makes us different from our friends and from our former roles in friendships. We need to confide in our friends, trying to strike a delicate balance between our needs and theirs. We need their support and understanding, although at times we pull back from them because of relapses and isolative tendencies. We need friends to be flexible and not take some of the things we do personally. We become needier, able to do things less often, more preoccupied with how we are feeling, and sometimes we are reluctant to reach out to others. Friendships become pressured and strained. Like other relationships, friendships may be strengthened in the process or may be lost, unable to withstand the changes.

Here is what some PWCs have said about friendships:

> My friends have been real supportive of me. They take good care of me and yell at me to rest and take care of myself. Most of my friends are in the health care field; they are used to health issues being a part of their lives.

> I have found out who my real friends are. There are those who understand and those who want me to push too hard.

> My personal life has gone down the tubes, so to speak. I was dating and now feel unable to do that. I find that people are so afraid of catching something from me. I am upset most of the time.

> I lost most of my friends and feel devastated.

Most of us experience a combination of reactions from others. Special efforts at communication are required, presenting a problem when our energy is limited. Friendship becomes a balancing act between their needs and ours, which have grown to astounding proportions. The test of a friendship is its degree of flexibility—how well it can withstand change and allow for communication about what both parties are experiencing. Can our friends accept our limitations without judgment? Do they accept that we are ill despite obvious signs? Will they accept us even when we're at our worst? Will our friends love us even though it's difficult for us to love ourselves? Friends may disappear, stick with us unconditionally or withstand only the early stages of the illness, distancing themselves when CFIDS continues to linger. Each friendship is different, but one constant remains: it is essential to talk with each of our friends not only about CFIDS but about the effects it is having on the friendship. Doing this will not assure longevity of the relationship but it's our best shot. Readjustment and rebalancing are necessary over time if the friendship is to survive.

Chapter 9

———————◆———————

C-Kids: CFIDS in Children

CHILDREN AS WELL AS ADULTS may get CFIDS. Although it is commonly believed that the majority of patients are adults, it is speculated that the incidence of CFIDS in children equals that of adults but is underdiagnosed in the under-twenty population. CFIDS is especially difficult for kids because they have not yet fully developed their capabilities and identities and often don't have a sense yet of what is "normal" for them. Young children with an insidious onset of CFIDS haven't yet "become accustomed to the way they think" and may not even understand CFIDS as an external event, reports David Bell, M.D., a pediatrician and CFIDS researcher who is the expert on CFIDS in children.

CFIDS is rare in children under the age of five. Onset of CFIDS in children ages five through twelve is generally gradual, whereas onset at or after puberty is more common and more likely to be sudden. Unlike CFIDS in adults, Bell finds that the numbers of male and female children with CFIDS are about equal. He reports that about 75% experience an acute onset with infection whereas 25% have a more gradual onset of symptoms. Because those with a gradual onset are more likely to remain undiagnosed, these figures may be somewhat inaccurate.

Since symptoms of CFIDS in children differ from those in adults, Bell has developed a different set of diagnostic criteria.

Six of these eight symptoms must have been present constantly or intermittently for at least six months:

1. Fatigue

2. Neurologic complaints

3. Headache

4. Sore throat

5. Arthralgia (joint pain)

6. Myalgia (muscle pain)

7. Abdominal pain

8. Lymphatic pain

Alternatively, the criteria are satisfied when five of the above symptoms are present along with two of the following three:

1. Rash

2. Fever, chills and/or night sweats

3. Eye pain and/or photophobia (light sensitivity)
   (*The CFIDS Chronicle*, January/February 1989, p. 7).

Bell has reported immune disregulation findings similar to those in adults. Many children with CFIDS have histories of allergies and other infections. In some cases their CFIDS symptoms continue into adulthood.

Children generally have more symptoms and more varied symptoms than do adults, and may have different ones each day. Children often have difficulty describing their symptoms, especially neurological problems, including attention deficit, dizziness and disequilibrium, memory impairment, word-finding problems, impaired visual/spatial perception and, less frequently, seizure-like episodes. Emotional symptoms such as depression and rapid mood changes are difficult for children to understand and manage. In addition, children with CFIDS may experience nightmares and sleep disorders, weight loss, weakness, lack of interest in work or play, behavioral disorders, and exhaustion following physical exercise, according to Byron Hyde, M.D. Hyde feels that many children remain undiagnosed because adults do not believe they are ill and that the resulting frustration is the cause of some child and adolescent suicides. These children are experiencing considerable trauma: CFIDS symptoms, coupled with the disbelief or misunderstanding of others and an inability to perform adequately to meet others' expectations.

Those with milder symptoms and/or an acute onset are more likely to recover spontaneously, according to Bell. Children with allergies and/or a more gradual onset of symptoms generally remain ill longer and are less likely to recover, although they may improve slowly over time. However, this information is speculative and has not been studied systematically.

Parents and school personnel may have difficulty understanding these symptoms and the resulting behavior and mood changes. Often the undiagnosed child is perceived as being resistant, seeking secondary gains of illness, or being lazy, school-phobic, neurotic, psychotic, or having learning disabilities. Or the child may be misdiagnosed with another illness based on individual symptom patterns.

Neurocognitive testing may reveal a characteristic pattern, according to Bell, and special learning plans should be developed by school personnel if necessary. Academic performance may be significantly affected; grades typically go down and school attendance is often spotty (October 1988).

Family disruption may be significant. Children with CFIDS are often unable to participate in family activities. If the child has not been properly diagnosed, the family is unable to understand changes in health and behavior. Even with a correct diagnosis, the inability to perform chores and to participate in family outings causes strain. Siblings resent the preferential treatment of the ill child, and the ill child may blame him or herself for the illness and feel like a burden to the family. The ill child may feel "abnormal" and "different" from peers and other family members, a considerable blow to identity formation and self-esteem.

A woman whose young daughter has CFIDS called me to arrange a consultation, saying that her daughter Lisa, a fourth grader, was experiencing adjustment problems, as were other family members. Formerly an active, vivacious child, Lisa had begun to tire easily and to become reclusive. She retreated to her room for long naps directly after school each day, awakened to eat dinner, then returned to bed and slept until the next morning. Lisa had become "overly sensitive to everything and anything," according to her mother. She snapped at others with little or no provocation. She no longer participated in family activities and had no energy to do her chores, causing resent-ment among her siblings. The need for family counseling was clearly demonstrated so that all could learn to cope appro-priately, problem solve, and adapt to Lisa's illness.

An intelligent, perceptive fourteen-year-old PWC has asked me to refer to him as "John Doe." He and his parents describe numerous symptoms; most prominent are fatigue, depression, and cognitive impairment. John is unable to attend school and is bored at home despite homebound instruction. He is isolated from his peers and uncomfortably dependent upon his parents, from whom he is trying to individuate—a normal develop-mental task. John is often unsure how much of his emotional turmoil is CFIDS-related and how much is attributable to typi-cal adolescent development. Having experienced bouts of severe depression and suicidal ideations (with several suicide attempts), John wrote about his feelings:

Mirror Image

It was dark, not an ordinary dark but more of a heavy dark. He shivered, yet it wasn't cold at least not to him. It is here that the sensation came. The sensation of danger. It always startled him even though its presence was known. Panicking him into paranoia, the presence upset him. It upset him with its chaoticness and havoc. It was there, although he couldn't define it, but it was there. His thoughts always merged and the colors ran together. Leaving him threatened by defense-lessness. He liked the aloneness of this play, blocked off from the world. He was scared, and needed help. But something blocked off the given, the presence blocked it off. Using the tasteful aloneness to make him not want the help. The presence was in control and he was torn between what he needed and what he wanted. He needed help, he wanted aloneness. So help never came, and he sank deeply into his mind, searching for what it didn't matter. What he found left him pale. For in the far reaches of his thoughts was a mirror. In the mirror was an illness, the illness was himself, his darker self. He screamed, maybe help would come now.

Once diagnosed with CFIDS, John began seeing a helpful and sensitive physician who has referred him to a psychologist. John has made considerable progress physically and emotionally, but he remains ill and experiences frequent relapses.

CFIDS in children can be a heartbreaking event for them and for their families. Parents are virtually helpless as the illness runs its unpredictable course. An accurate diagnosis and treatment by a well-informed, compassionate physician are essential. Family education and communication are extremely important, and counseling is often helpful. Although a child's emotional, social, and academic growth may be adversely affected, children are marvelously adaptable, and often their health will improve over time.

PART III

CFIDS: What to Do

Chapter 10

◆

The Medical Profession

Men of the cure have been more cruel than the disease.
                    Miguel de Cervantes, *Don Quixote*

            What's up, Doc?
                    Bugs Bunny

THOSE OF US WITH CHRONIC ILLNESSES often get negative reactions from a medical community that deals primarily with acute problems. We fall through the cracks of medicine. When we are ill, we are expected to do one of two things: get well or die. Yet we do neither, nor do all of us respond in the same ways to treatment. We are a difficult lot to work with, and so are many of our doctors. The inability of medicine to deal productively with illness lacking a known cause and a specific remedy is apparent in the stories told by patients.

Some PWCs have been fortunate in finding good medical care, but many doctor-shop for years. Those who have been ill long-term, and even some whose onset has been more recent, may have seen 10 or 20 doctors before finding one who could diagnose the problem correctly. Some of our symptoms are those typically ascribed to neurotic, depressed people who are accused of enjoying medical and social attention for their ailments. That there are so many of us with similar symptoms (which developed over a period of time during which we didn't know anyone else in the world was similarly afflicted) suggests an organic illness. Doctors usually form diagnoses based upon laboratory tests and physical examinations. Since there is still no test for CFIDS and because many of the symptoms we describe are not apparent in a physical exam, the diagnosis of CFIDS requires special understanding and knowledge on the part of the physician. To diagnose CFIDS, the physician must be familiar with the diagnostic criteria, listen carefully to the patient's description, take a thorough history, and order tests to rule out other illnesses. Unfortunately, this process takes a lot of time— a commodity that is in short supply in most doctors' offices. The time problem is a serious dilemma because insurance companies have largely taken over the political realm of medicine. As a result many doctors are now seeing larger numbers of patients to make up for reduced fee allowances from insurance companies. At a time when patients are becoming more consumer-oriented and insisting that their needs be met, doctors are finding it increasingly difficult to spend more time with their patients. This serious problem is not easily solved.

Many of the patients who consult me report that they have been diagnosed on the basis of Epstein-Barr antibody panel results. Probably many more who reported similar symptoms but "failed" the blood test were told they were fine (or crazy) and sent home. Many doctors are still testing for EBV alone and diagnosing CFIDS inappropriately on that basis, rather than applying the now-accepted diagnostic criteria. Although we cannot expect doctors to be aware of all the nuances of every current health problem, we can expect them to be attentive, thorough, and willing to explore.

Conventional medicine is challenged by today's medical consumers. Sources of patient dissatisfaction with allopathic (mainstream) medicine are many. First, allopathic medicine has become a high-tech maze, offering sophisticated equipment and procedures with both benefits and risks. Overreliance on technology and data alone results in decreased attention to the individual patient. Second, medicine has become big business, and insurance companies are now sufficiently powerful to exert financial control over the medical profession, keeping it on a tight leash. Third, patients are becoming increasingly disgruntled with the degree of medical specialization today and irritated about being shuffled among specialists while never being given an opportunity to present the whole picture or to be treated as a whole person. Fourth, the public has become more consumer-oriented, more aware of its needs and rights, and thus more demanding of time, attention, explanations, and alternatives in medical matters. Fifth, patients have become more openly resentful toward what they perceive as cursory and/or condescending treatment when their complaints are trivialized by their doctors. Sixth, medical consumers are now examining options, recognizing that allopathic physicians are not demi-gods practicing the only valid type of medicine, but simply one alternative among the types of health care available.

CONCEPTS OF ILLNESS AND WELLNESS

In our society, illness is viewed as something that happens to a person as a result of a germ or an accident. The body is broken and needs to be fixed. Something has gone wrong at the biological level. But illness is not simply an interaction between a "bad" germ and a "good" body. When exposed to a germ, some become ill and others do not. The larger picture must be considered: genetic makeup; environmental conditions; nutrition; our thoughts, beliefs, and feelings; social interactions; addictions; emotional stress and pain; abuse of our bodies; how we live our lives. Why do some people who are exposed to a germ become ill while others do not?

The very concepts of illness and wellness are poorly understood. "We know health well in its absence," wrote Andrew Weil. Apart from being merely the absence of illness, however, the term wellness connotes a harmony of mind, body, and spirit, and an appropriate style of living. It also connotes self-care—proper nutrition, rest, and exercise. Attention to these aspects of health have generated unfortunate health fads: we seek to purchase magic remedies in our instant-fix-oriented society. But the wellness we seek cannot be purchased or easily achieved.

One mistake I have made in my quest for wellness is having the unrealistic expectation of too much too soon. I continued to pursue an instant solution, unwilling to accept the reasonable approach of achieving balance in my life by budgeting my energy, learning to be less rushed and pressured, and making gradual changes in the way I lived as I continued to explore and experiment with treatment options. We tend to think that there's *one* thing we should do, or a specific approach or philosophy to follow that will make us well, and we look for someone who can tell us what it is. If we can't find an allopath who can do it, we look for someone outside mainstream medicine who can. To seek medical care that will augment the healing process is sensible; to expect a magical cure is not.

THE SPECIAL PROBLEMS OF CHRONIC ILLNESS

> Wildly expensive medical care has made little advance against chronic and catastrophic illness while becoming steadily more impersonal, more intrusive.
> M. Ferguson, *The Aquarian Conspiracy*

Doctors have a better success rate with acute illnesses than with chronic ones. Chronically ill patients have ongoing needs that present special challenges for health care providers. The chronically ill often do not look sick and tend to have unpredictable changes in health. We become experts on our illnesses and challenge our physicians. Doctors and other medical personnel often cannot comprehend what they can't see or measure. We claim to be ill, but our symptoms keep changing and most aren't obvious to other people. In requesting treatment for a problem that's invisible and difficult to define, we often feel rejected by the medical system on which we depend. In our frustrating quest to be treated as sane people with a continuing, crazy-making illness, we alternately seek treatment from a system that doesn't welcome us, or we become hopeless.

Of course doctors prefer to work with easier-to-diagnose and easier-to-treat illnesses. Doctors are trained to cure people and that's what they like to do. When they can't fix what's wrong, they become frustrated; their egos are threatened. Once a series of expensive diagnostic tests has produced negative results, the patient may be referred elsewhere for what is then viewed as a "psychosomatic" (in an incorrect, pejorative sense) illness. The temptation to dump us on some other specialty such as psychiatry is great.

We are a huge inconvenience to practitioners who have the attitude that any illness involving unexplained symptoms and normal results on lab tests is not to be taken too seriously. Those of us with chronic illnesses *are* pains in the ass to our doctors. We don't get better, we don't go away, we just keep coming back with the same old complaints and additional new ones. We tell our doctors how awful we feel, and if they take us seriously, they have only two attitudinal choices: to feel badly about how little they have to offer us by way of treatment, or to harden themselves against their failure to make us well. The latter is a survival mechanism, born of the doctor's need to be a hero, a fixer, a curer of ills, and to see anything less as a failure. We present a challenge and a threat.

Most doctors don't state their frustration openly but demonstrate it in more subtle ways which make their patients unhappy. Patients with CFIDS often feel rejected and neglected by their physicians; they either continue with their doctors while harboring resentment against them, or they seek medical attention elsewhere. Switching from one doctor to another or fragmenting care among several doctors is common among PWCs.

When the case definition for CFIDS was finally published in March 1988, affording us a legitimate status among the chronically ill, Marc Iverson, president of The CFIDS Association of Charlotte, North Carolina, wrote an article called "The Politics of CFIDS: A Salute for Some, An 'I Told You So' for Others."

> For good reason, many of us harbor feelings of anger and bitterness about the insensitive way these [non-believing] physicians treated us for so many years. Too many doctors . . . simply did not *listen* to us. With great arrogance, they con-

cluded that just because they could not understand our illness (and their technology could not detect it) it did not exist and must therefore be 'in our heads' (i.e. 'psychosomatic'). How ironic it is that neuropsychological testing and MRI brain scans seem to indicate that for many CFIDS patients the illness literally *is* in their heads! For those of us who endured years of patronizing attitudes, demeaning remarks, and humiliating treatment at the hands of all-knowing, closed-minded physicians, I say to the guilty parties, damn it, you failed us and you failed yourselves. Most of us have emerged from this experience with our self-respect intact and our perspective on life enhanced. I wonder if this is true of those physicians who selfishly washed their hands of our difficult cases and dishonored their noble profession. (*The CFIDS Chronicle,* April 1988)

Doctors would like us to cooperate by getting well, and we'd love to comply, not for the sake of their egos but for the sake of our health. However, physicians must learn to treat chronic illnesses without blaming us for remaining ill or themselves for not curing us.

CFIDS PATIENTS TALK
ABOUT MEDICAL TREATMENT

Most initial doctor visits involve recitations of symptoms and the inevitable question from not-yet-diagnosed CFIDS patients, "What's wrong with me?" Usually their inquiries are met with a variety of discouraging responses, including accusations of hypochondriasis, inappropriate lifestyles, and inability to handle stress, and neurosis. Or their complaints are dismissed as menopause, laziness, a "bug," or generalized anxiety.

Some patients report helpful responses from their doctors:

I don't know. Let's run some tests and see if we can find the problem.

I've seen a lot of people with these symptoms lately. I'm not sure what's causing them.

It sounds to me like you have CFS/CFIDS. I don't really know much about it, but I'll see what I can find out. *Or:* I'll refer you to someone who has experience with treatment of this illness.

I can help you with CFIDS, but I can't cure you.

Other patients report upsetting experiences:

I've been sent to a separate specialist for each of my symptoms. None of them understands that all these things seem to be connected. They won't listen when I tell them this is all one illness.

I was tested by a psychologist [neuropsychological evaluation]. He was mad at me; he said a third grader could do things on the test that I couldn't do. He thought I was making it all up, that I just didn't want to work any more . . . . I had a cushy job that I loved, and I was making a lot of money. Why would I want to stop? And my doctor believed everything this guy reported to him; he didn't believe me.

The nurse in my doctor's office said, "You must know you're causing these problems yourself." I told her I was driving in a familiar street and just got lost. I didn't know where I was, and that was scary. She acted like I made it up. I told my doctor about it . . . but he didn't listen to me and didn't understand.

My doctor finally told me what's wrong. The advice I got was, "Just adapt to it. Rest a lot. Learn to manage stress. Persevere and be patient."

Such advice as, "Just accept the illness and go on with your life" is easier given than followed. It implies falsely that no treatment is available. Patients come away quite discouraged. Some give up passively and others decide to fight, to educate themselves about available alternatives.

PWCs have expressed anger, bitterness, and distrust toward the medical profession in general and certain doctors in particular. However, many have indicated that they found at least one physician with whose attitude and treatment approach they were pleased. Patients have indicated the qualities in a physician they deem most valuable: competence, honesty, warmth, concern, willingness to listen carefully to the patient, being down-to-earth, spending adequate time with the patient, and a willingness to explore treatment alternatives. Patients greatly appreciate doctors who are willing to take the extra time to answer questions and offer explanations. Many patients have indicated being most satisfied with doctors who themselves had CFIDS or other chronic illnesses, or whose staff members, wives or family members had CFIDS. Usually these doctors were more likely to understand what their patients were experiencing.

TYPES OF MEDICAL PRACTICE

Not all doctors practice the same type of medicine. In this section various approaches to medical practice are discussed. I am not advocating any particular form of treatment but simply describing options.

Physical approaches to healing

Allopathy   Most mainstream doctors in the United States practice allopathic medicine. Allopathic treatment relies upon the use of pharmaceuticals and technology, which are often effective for acute medical problems such as trauma, acute illness, and repair or replacement of joints and organs. Sophisticated technology allows us access to the internal workings of our bodies, in many cases with noninvasive procedures. Many allopathic doctors are sensitive, caring, and open-minded, but others have become rigid, closed to new ideas, and disenchanted with the practice of medicine, because medical insurance companies are increasingly directing the practice of medicine. Sara Reynolds, M.D., adds, "Unfortunately, many physicians have learned from sad experience to beware of the apparent 'doctor-shopper' who goes from office to office 'til he or she gets the [desired] treatment or medicine."

Doctors often seem to be more preoccupied with their machinery than with the health of their patients. Studies have shown that touch is very important in mobilizing healing, but technology pushes doctors further away from their patients. The awe in which we hold hard science leads to a reliance on objective measures that is not necessarily in the best interests of the patient. Tests are most productive if used in conjunction with other findings.

The allopathic model draws artificial distinctions between illnesses of the mind and those of the body and tends to enforce the unfortunate notion of mind-body duality. The concept of the mindbody as an integrated entity is an old one that is coming back into favor. By ignoring the role of consciousness in the patient's states of wellness and illness the allopathic doctor adds to the distance between doctor and patient, and the two often fail to interact well.

Allopathic medicine is often accused of falling short in dealing with chronic illness. Drugs can offer symptomatic relief, but deeper causes of chronic problems are less easily detected or treated. Allopathy has also been criticized for a lack of attention to preventive medicine and health maintenance, although patients often do not follow advice regarding health maintenance. Fortunately many allopaths—usually the family practitioner or the internist—are attentive and responsive to their patients and treat them holistically.

Allopathic medicine has both strengths and shortcomings. " . . . [A]lthough disenchanted with establishment medicine," wrote Locke and Colligan, "we must be aware of the danger of turning wholeheartedly to other forms of treatment. The risks of alternative practices are in some cases ignored or minimized" (1986, p. 185). Sara Reynolds, M.D., comments: "Unfortunately, when anything is touted as miraculous or seems 'too good to be true' it probably is. Most allopathic [treatment] is based on scientific evidence. Most other therapy is anecdotal but may be valid."

Osteopathy Although this branch of healing is theoretically based on the structural aspects of the body (bones, muscles, and joints), osteopathy increasingly has come to resemble allopathy in the use of pharmacological drugs and other interventions. Osteopathic manipulation is used as a treatment approach (but not the sole approach to medical problems, a criticism leveled at chiropractic practice. Do not confuse the two!) Doctors trained in osteopathy (D.O.s) often pay more attention than allopaths to the whole patient and many stress the body's own healing powers.

Allopathic and osteopathic medical facilities are usually separate; however, the two types of medical degrees (M.D. and D.O.) are legally equivalent in all states. It becomes increasingly evident that sound medical practice and a positive relationship with patients rather than the type of diploma are the truly relevant aspects of quality medical care, and cooperation between the allopath and osteopath would be beneficial to practitioners and patients alike.

Homeopathy   Homeopathic doctors seek to treat the whole body, to balance and to strengthen it, and to identify symptom patterns in each patient. Homeopaths emphasize the individual and the individual's manifestations of illness, seeking to stimulate healing by tapping the body's healing powers rather than by simply medicating symptoms. They do not rely heavily on lab tests to produce diagnoses; labels are not considered important. Rather than treating with pharmaceuticals, homeopathy works by isolating substances that, when administered, tend to produce symptoms like those the patient is experiencing. These substances are then highly diluted and administered so that the body will react against them, thus fighting the symptoms. The theory is that a small amount of what caused the problem will fix it. A few scientific studies have been conducted, but it remains speculative why this approach is successful in some cases.

At present, some disenchanted mainstream physicians are considering alternatives and some are "converting" to homeopathy. They feel that allopathic medicine has been ineffective in combating chronic and degenerative diseases, which abound today. They stress the need for prevention and education.

The practice of homeopathy is regarded with suspicion by most mainstream medical practitioners, and the AMA has taken an exclusionary view of homeopaths. Homeopathic treatment is quite expensive and is not generally covered by medical insurance.

Naturopathy   Naturopaths believe in the ability of nature to heal. They focus on the body's innate healing ability and on curative properties of certain natural substances in the environment, such as plants and molds, which are the origins of many pharmaceutical products. Naturopathy seems to be gaining in popularity but remains unaccepted by most people as a viable approach to medical treatment. Although the healing power of nature is certainly real, naturopaths lack a consistent, shared methodical approach to treatment and some of their practices are unproven. Some PWCs have reported excellent results with naturopathic healers while others have not been helped.

Traditional Chinese medicine   We usually associate Chinese medicine with herbal preparations, acupuncture, t'ai chi, and qigong, with mysticism and healing masters. Ironically, many regard traditional Chinese medicine as a fad, part of "New Age" medicine, but it is an ancient practice steeped in tradition. It takes an integrated approach, more subtle than that of Western medicine, combining physical and "spiritual" or "mental" healing.

The unifying concept behind the tradition is the belief that the body has a number of meridians (circuits) that conduct energy throughout the body. Symptoms result from a blockage in these meridians, and healing is directed at removing the blockages so that energy can once again flow freely. The individual, rather than a particular illness, is the focus of treatment. Symptoms are viewed in terms of the functioning of the entire body, and the treatment goal is to locate and correct energy imbalances that manifest themselves as symptoms.

Acupuncture is a treatment process in which fine needles, sometimes along with heat, electricity, oils, or lasers, are inserted at various trigger points along the body's meridians. The energy points chosen depend on the nature of the patient's complaint or the treatment goal. Some PWCs report that acupuncture restores energy, improves vestibular functioning, and enhances feelings of well-being. While its mechanism of action is not fully understood, acupuncture is believed to stimulate the body's production of enkephalin (beta endorphin) and serotonin, creating changes in mood and sleep. Although many in the West view it as a radical or new treatment, acupuncture has been practiced for centuries and may become a standard component of integrated medical treatment in the future. Acupressure is similar to acupuncture, but instead of needles, a trained massage practitioner applies pressure to certain trigger points on the body's surface.

Chinese medicine takes a long-term preventive approach which is also helpful for chronic illness. Western medicine is acknowledged by practitioners of Chinese medicine to be more appropriate for trauma and acute illness. A combination of Eastern and Western medicine may be the accepted treatment modality of the twenty-first century.

Ayurvedic medicine One of the holistic approaches to medicine, ayurvedic philosophy and medical practice originates in India. It focuses on a wholesome lifestyle, incorporating diet, herbal preparations, massage, meditation, and behavior. The whole person rather than the disease label is the focus of treatment. Treatment is aimed at producing feelings of well-being and is claimed to be helpful for health maintenance and the treatment of minor disorders.

Other types of "physical" healing Many other healing approaches, including chiropractic and nutritional therapy, are eyed with suspicion by the medical community and society in general. Despite considerable controversy, many patients claim to have been helped by "unorthodox" methods. Each treatment has its advantages and limitations, and the patient's belief system plays a large part in determining the success of any treatment. The availability and growing popularity of alternative approaches indicate that there is no one correct approach to medical treatment. The role of nutrient supplementation and diet as an adjunct to a treatment program is discussed further in Chapter 11.

Mental or "spiritual" approaches to healing

Positive thinking, faith healing, and medicine men In the growing movement of patient empowerment and the belief in the healing properties of the human body, positive motivation toward healing and wellness is respected and considered potent. This discussion includes such diverse healing systems as shamanism, Christian Science, and folk healing, since in all these cases intervention is believed to be a supernatural, or at least superhuman, phenomenon. Generally regarded with disfavor as being superstitious and ritualistic, such approaches are oriented toward the intervention of forces beyond the usual range of human understanding and the limitations of our techno- logical and cultural beliefs. The individual's faith in the method is the basis of its success. Skeptics abound, especially in our culture in which science and logic are highly valued. By contrast, in these healing systems illness may be seen as the result of inappropriate or negative thinking on the part of the individual, or as the result of some external supernatural force. The key ingredient is faith—in the method, in the healer, in some sort of divine intervention. Healing rituals in communities that accept and believe in them apparently produce positive results. The group or community support, and the individual's spiritual belief are thought to be the potent ingredients in such healing practices.

In choosing treatment for a ruptured appendix, the need for surgical intervention is clearly demonstrable. An interaction between an intangible illness and an unobservable intervention, however, encourages skepticism even when successful results are obtained. The practices of prayer, imagery, belief in supernatural or invisible, innate healing sources, or any type of spiritual medicine is alien to our culture. Although we tend to believe in the "power of positive thinking," we have difficulty believing that it can truly help healing to take place. Can faith and belief transcend and overcome physical symptoms? If not, how can we explain the apparent success of these methods in many cases? We are skeptical of such procedures as hypnosis and guided imagery, but less so when technology such as biofeedback is introduced to demonstrate scientifically that something measurable is happening.

"We must be receptive to possibilities that science has not yet grasped, or we will miss them," wrote Bernie Siegel in *Love, Medicine and Miracles*. "It's absurd not to use treatments that work, just because we don't understand them." Joan Borysenko, too, in *Minding the Body, Mending the Mind*, is open to such alternative approaches. "We are entering a new level in the scientific understanding of mechanisms by which faith, belief, and imagination can actually unlock the mysteries of healing." Emotions and beliefs exert a direct influence on the brain and thus on the immune system, thereby facilitating healing. However, most experts agree that a superficial belief system—one that is based on what one would like to believe, but is not internalized—will be ineffective in creating positive change.

Psychology and psychiatry Although these fields are attaining more realistic and legitimate status in the mind of the public, the need for therapy is often as suspect as its practice. Mental health or behavioral health practitioners vary in approach, education, training, and personal style. Although therapy is not a panacea, it has practical application in many situations. The general goals of therapy include personal growth, insight, behavior change, enhancement of self-esteem, problem solving, and emotional support. Such issues may require only short-term therapy, while more complex, deep-seated issues may require long-term treatment. In many cases, the family of the PWC should be involved in therapy. Families have great difficulty accepting change, especially when former roles can no longer be filled by the PWC.

In my experience as a psychologist working with PWCs, I find that in most cases brief intervention is sufficient. Those who have difficulty accepting the diagnosis and limitations and those who resist modifying their activity levels and lifestyles are cause for particular concern. Denial of the illness is a natural stage in working toward acceptance, but those who become stuck in this stage may require intense therapeutic intervention to move beyond it. A PWC may have issues of long standing that are compounded and magnified by chronic illness. Such issues may involve former roles (especially for those who have been overly responsible for others, neglecting self-care), family of origin, financial concerns and attitudes, relationship problems, and low self-esteem. Working through these while coping with CFIDS-related concerns can be a lengthy but helpful process.

Although psychological counseling can hardly be considered a curative modality for an invading virus, it helps in the treatment of primarily physiological illnesses by addressing adjustment issues and mobilizing innate healing potential. Physical and psychological treatments should be highly integrated.

Healthy Suspician

Quacks and charlatans probably exist in all types of medical practice—physical, mental, and spiritual. Perhaps some approaches invite more scams than others, but none is exempt. A certain level of suspicion is healthy—we must not accept all new therapies blindly—but we should also guard against total rigidity and blind rejection of anything new or unusual. Any tool that minimizes helplessness and maximizes hopefulness is doing something helpful, even if we cannot demonstrate how or why.

Alternative treatment approaches vary widely in success rates, and many of their claims are probably unfounded. Additionally, many systems lack credentialing organizations and accredited or recognized training institutions. Often there are considerable variations in practice. Individual practitioners of the same type of medicine are often radically different from one another, not only in personality but in theory, approach, and cost. Medical insurance companies do not usually pay for any treatments considered by them to be "experimental." Unfortunately, with CFIDS there is no standard treatment program and so all interventions are considered experimental.

Treatment modalities range from beneficial to harmless to dangerous—and many are quite expensive. An outbreak of a new illness or increased attention to an existing one will invite the development and sale of various new substances and treatments. Such a flurry of new miracle approaches is cause for careful, wary consideration. Safety claims may be fabricated, especially when products are touted as "natural." (I can think of many natural substances, like cow dung and arsenic, that I would not care to ingest.) Any claims that a particular treatment program cures CFIDS or helps all PWCs is bogus; so far no treatment can claim such a track record.

TOWARD A NEW CONCEPT OF HEALTH AND HEALING

Developing a positive doctor-patient relationship

> We have oversold the benefits of technology and external manipulations; we have undersold the importance of human relationships and the complexity of nature.
>
> M. Ferguson, *The Aquarian Conspiracy*

One flaw in medical training is the lack of education in communication skills. Doctors are confronted daily with the fears and insecurities of their patients. The doctor's communication skills can increase or decrease this fear and confusion. Too often the communication is abrupt and cursory, leaving the patient with unanswered questions, assumptions, and new fears which may negatively affect the treatment outcome. Many doctors tend to give orders rather than offer explanations. For them, "difficult patients" are often those who ask questions, ask to participate in their health care, and expect that the physician will work with them toward a mutually satisfying outcome. Those doctors who demand patient compliance, ignore input from their patients, and act too busy to care are "difficult doctors." Patients and doctors should ask each other more questions, both for a more accurate assessment of the case and to help the patient become a better-informed, more cooperative (rather than compliant) participant.

We want doctors to be something more than mechanics. We demand that they pay attention to our concerns and treat us with compassion as well as competence—a lot to ask, but the only path to successful treatment. We appreciate new technology but abhor its overuse. Treatment of the whole patient is essential—not just test results, or an isolated symptom or body part, but the whole human being. Such progress requires a team approach and the education of doctors in such areas as communication skills, alternative approaches to healing and medicine, exercise, and nutrition. All healing is scientific, according to Bernie Siegel, M.D., even when we cannot explain how the healing occurs.

It is time to discard permanently the antiquated concept of mind-body duality and to use the term "psychosomatic" in its *true* sense, an acknowledgment that the integrated system called the mindbody experiences the illness. "The placebo is proof that there is no real separation between mind and body," wrote Norman Cousins:

> Illness is always an interaction among both. It can begin in the mind and affect the body, or it can begin in the body and affect the mind, both of which are served by the same bloodstream. Attempts to treat most mental diseases as though they were completely free of physical causes and attempts to treat most bodily diseases as though the mind were in no way involved must be considered archaic in the light of new evidence about the way the human body functions. (1979, pp. 56–57)

Empathizing with patients is said to present risk for the physician. We do not ask physicians to ignore their own needs for objectivity and distance but simply to meet us halfway. Bernie Siegel, M.D., believes that doctors are destined to fail as mechanics but have much to offer as empathetic counselors, teachers, and healers.

The power of touch should not be underestimated in the practice of medicine. Human touch brings healer and patient closer, counteracts some of the "cold" effects of modern medical technology, and conveys warmth and caring, important elements in healing. Massage, acupuncture, and acupressure are healing modalities that involve touch. Some physicians make it a practice to touch each patient during an examination or consultation.

Effective verbal communication, too, will help to bridge the gap. Patients fare better when procedures are explained, when they feel they are listened to, when they work together with the doctor in choosing the course of medical treatment. In my experience as a mediator I have found that people who participate in a decision-making process are more likely to comply with terms they have helped to develop. The same principle applies to consumers of health care, who are more likely to follow a treatment regimen they have played a part in selecting.

Patients and doctors each have responsibilities in their relationship. A true partnership between doctor and patient combines the perceptions and strengths of both based on a foundation of communication, trust, and mutual participation.

Responsibilities of the patient Physicians are experts in the field of medicine but are human beings first. Arthur Schimelfenig, Ph.D., said in a lecture to the Greater Phoenix Area CFIDS Support Group, "If you expect your physician to pull you out of this, forget it. You're the best treatment you've got. Use your doctors to help you."

As a patient, some of the things you are responsible for are:

1. Identifying and stating your needs. If you have a complaint about medical care, bring it to the attention of your doctor in a straightforward, not critical or accusatory manner. Complaining isn't productive, but direct requests often are. Learn to communicate assertively.

2. Ask questions when you need information about your illness, prognosis, medications, or other treatment options. Specific questions will generate clearer answers. Recognize that the answer to many of your questions will be, "I don't know." Because many doctors are uncomfortable saying this, you might get a circuitous answer. If you do, ask a more specific question or say, "Is this something you can look into further?" or "Do you know if any research is being done in this area?"

3. Become aware of the role you are playing as a patient. Are you playing the role of the dependent child, expecting your doctor to be the magic, healing parent? Most effective is an adult-to-adult relationship based on mutual respect and your need for a competent, caring medical professional—not a parent.

4. Differentiate between cooperation and obedience. A cooperative patient works helpfully along with the physician; an obedient one simply does what she or he is told without questioning. Cooperation gets the best results in the long run, although obedience may earn pats on the head.

5. Be well informed about CFIDS. Share information with your doctor, making it clear that your purpose is to discuss the issues, not to tell your doctor how to practice medicine. Physicians can't keep up with every new development in medicine but should be willing to consider new information presented by patients.

6. Be a well-informed consumer of medical care. Shop carefully for your experts; you're the customer. Question your doctor about rates for various services. Of course, your decision to see a particular doctor should not hinge solely (or even primarily) on costs, but you have the right to know up front what the charges will be. Comparison-shop when filling prescriptions. Consider generic drug prescriptions (but be aware that in some cases generics are of lesser quality; talk with your doctor and pharmacist about the pros and cons of generics).

7. Keep careful track of your appointments and give 24-hour notice (except in cases of emergency) if you cannot keep an appointment. Arrive on time. If the doctor is habitually late, discuss this problem not with the staff but with the doctor, who is ultimately responsible for scheduling.

8. Be organized. Maintain lists of (a) your symptoms and concerns, (b) any questions you have, (c) all medications

you are taking, and (d) any medications to which you have had unusual or adverse reactions in the past. If you have consulted other doctors in the past, keep copies of your medical records, including lab test results, and make them available to your new physician(s).

9. Listen attentively to what the doctor says during your discussions and take notes. Ask questions until you are sure you understand the answers. Information that makes sense at the time can be difficult to remember later. You might consider bringing someone to appointments with you to corroborate or expand on your history, offer observations, and clarify information if necessary.

10. Recognize that medicine is not a hard science, and that diagnoses and treatment plans are judgment calls based on objective and subjective information. If you still harbor the unrealistic expectation that the doctor's responsibility is to identify a single medical cure for a long-term illness, recognize that the problem is too complex for such a simple solution. The lifestyle modification that must accompany medical intervention is the responsibility of the patient.

11. Don't fake feeling better than you do just to please the doctor. Although doctors like their patients to get well, you are doing a disservice to your own treatment if you pretend. Your job isn't to be good, to please, or to meet unrealistic expectations of wellness. You have a responsibility to be honest.

12. If you need extra time with the doctor, request it when making your appointment. Expect to be charged for the additional time. If you are a new patient, tell the receptionist so when scheduling your appointment. And make sure the doctor is someone who is experienced in diagnosing and treating CFIDS.

13. If you are pleased with the medical treatment you are receiving, communicate your satisfaction to the doctor. Enumerate the qualities that are most valuable to you in

the care you are receiving. Specific praise is most helpful and gratifying to the recipient.

Responsibilities of the doctor

1. Jump off the pedestal. Let your patients know that you don't view yourself as omniscient. Accept that you cannot be totally in charge and in control at all times.

2. Talk to your patients. Tell them what you think; tell them you don't know or aren't sure when appropriate—that you don't have all the answers. Initially you may disappoint them, but in the long run you will be doing them (and yourself) a service. Offer explanations and information and explore alternatives with the patient.

3. Listen to your patients. If you don't understand, ask questions—without preconceived notions as to what the answers will be. Their statements will be at least as informative as their lab test results, and your willingness to listen demonstrates your caring.

4. Take your patients seriously. Patients often overhear doctors talking about them or other patients in a flippant manner. This behavior is insulting, hurtful, and trivializing. Please recognize that you are dealing with human beings, not cases. No one wants to be "the appendectomy in Room 402." Avoid the labels "somatizer," "hypochondriac," "neurotic," and "crock." All symptoms have origins, and all should be taken seriously. If you don't understand what's going on, say so, but don't dispute with the patient whether a "real" illness exists.

5. Avoid assuming a parental role that creates childlike dependence and ultimately resentment on the part of your patients. This type of dependency is dangerous, making you the responsible party and the patient the passive one.

6. Patients with chronic illnesses have special needs, ongoing ones. You may be unable to diagnose or treat their illnesses. If such is the case, tell them so and help them

decide what their next step is to be. Let the patient know you cannot effect a quick cure or alleviate all of their suffering but that you are available to them as a resource and a helper.

7. Recognize that some patients will return time after time without basic improvement. This is not your failure or theirs: it is a characteristic of the illness. It is natural to want your patients' health to improve with treatment and to be disappointed if there is no change or a negative one, but avoid making statements that cause the patient to feel guilty for a lack of progress. Assume that you are both doing the best you can and no one is to blame for a lack of improvement.

8. Keep an open mind about newly emerging concepts regarding CFIDS treatment. Patients with CFIDS have a strong network and will hear of various treatments that sound "far out," but such options should be considered if they are not likely to cause harm. Sara Reynolds, M.D., adds, "Don't criticize any treatment which appears helpful unless it is known to be detrimental in some way."

9. When a referral for psychological treatment is warranted, explain the purpose of the referral—support, neuropsychological evaluation, or help with problem solving, adjustment issues, stress management, coping skills, etc. If you make the referral with an inference that the illness is "all in the patient's head," you are using psychology/psychiatry as a dumping ground and will alienate the patient.

10. Your patients have emotional needs that are not separable from their medical needs. Although the physician need not play the therapist's role, it is important that patients be given support and understanding. Patients need to have their suffering acknowledged although it can't be "fixed." A simple statement such as "I realize this is really rough for you," can be of more help than most physicians realize. While the doctor is conceptualizing the disease, the patient is experiencing difficulty, confusion, and fear.

11. Offer your patients guidance in learning to take responsibility for their own care in terms of lifestyle modification (diet, exercise, etc.). Suggestions, explanation of rationale, and encouragement are helpful. Patients often feel "disciplined" (shamed or scolded) by their doctors, which reinforces dysfunctional parent-child roles. A preface such as "I know it's really hard to give up some of the things you really like, but ... " encourages the patient to perceive the suggestion as a source of positive motivation rather than an order. Patients are often fearful that their doctors will "yell at them" to promote compliance; empathetic guidance works better.

12. Show respect for your patients by keeping to your appointment schedule as closely as possible. It is demeaning to a patient to be kept waiting for long periods of time. In cases of emergency most patients will understand, but lateness on a regular basis is not acceptable. It may be necessary for you to discuss such chronic scheduling problems with your office staff.

13. Some of your CFIDS patients are more knowledgeable about their illness than you are. Many have read extensively, networked, and contacted support groups to obtain information. Allow patients to share this information with you.

CHOOSING A DOCTOR WISELY

The worst way to find a doctor is to consult the yellow pages for a name that sounds good or a location that is convenient. I wouldn't even choose a plumber this way.

Here are some suggestions for finding competent medical care:

✦ Consult your local CFIDS support group for a list of doctors who are experienced in treating CFIDS. Get referrals from other CFIDS patients or from doctors in whom you have confidence. You may need to see several types of specialists for treatment (e.g., internal medicine, allergy/

immunology, infectious disease, urology, endocrinology, and gastroenterology), but use a primary physician to consolidate and oversee treatment.

✦ Consult *The American Medical Directory: Physicians in the United States* in the reference section of your public library to get information about individual physicians, including type of practice, training, credentials, and board certification.

✦ Once you have chosen a candidate, ask if the doctor treats CFIDS and how long she or he spends with each new patient. If the answers are satisfactory, make an appointment to interview the doctor. You are in a "hiring" situation. Prepare pertinent questions in advance. Be aware of the validity of your needs.

✦ Use referrals and information about a doctor as a general guide, then trust your instincts to determine if you can work well with this person, if you feel a sense of trust and respect. Ask yourself these questions:
— Do I feel comfortable with this doctor? Is this someone in whom I can confide?
— Do I feel listened to and understood? Am I being given the doctor's full attention, free from distractions?
— Are there likely to be power struggles? Is this person abrupt or arrogant?
— Is this person knowledgeable about CFIDS and treatment options?
— Does this doctor have an open, accepting, positive attitude?
— Do we share the same treatment philosophy?
— Is a sense of hope being communicated to me?
— Is this person willing to admit uncertainty, to say "I don't know" when applicable?
— Do I have the sense that this doctor is interested in me as a person, not just a medical case?

No physician will get an A+ in every category. Decide which qualities are the most important; you won't find perfection! Don't expect inappropriate favors from the doctor, such as falsifications on insurance forms or frequent long telephone calls in place of office visits.

In some areas of the country, PWCs have been unable to find practitioners who are knowledgeable about CFIDS. As the medical community becomes better educated about CFIDS this problem will diminish. Currently these PWCs have few options: they can either educate a willing doctor or travel to a practitioner in another area.

IF YOU ARE DISSATISFIED WITH YOUR DOCTOR . . .

Many patients complain about poor doctor-patient communication. The highly motivated patient who addresses specific problem issues directly will probably obtain better results from the health care system.

First, examine your complaints or needs to determine if they are valid. If so, discuss the problem openly with the doctor, not a member of the staff. Do not accuse, attack, or make assumptions; this will put the doctor on the defensive, making it more difficult for the two of you to solve the problem and create a mutually satisfying therapeutic relationship. Make requests for change in a considerate, positive way, focusing on each specific problem and the desired outcome or solution options, and evaluate the doctor's response. Because most patients feel more comfortable grumbling to others than discussing problems directly with their doctors, your doctor may be surprised to hear of your dissatisfaction. Your doctor may have requests of you as well; try to listen objectively to assess their validity before reacting defensively.

If you can agree on changes to be made, allow a reasonable time for them to take place. If the problem is not corrected, you can persist or switch to another doctor. Once you have chosen another practitioner, obtain previous medical records or have them transferred.

If you have switched several times and are still dissatisfied, your expectations may be unrealistic. Perhaps no doctor can provide what you're seeking. However, do not compromise your values or reasonable standards. You should expect competent, compassionate, sensitive medical care and should not tolerate arrogance or indifference.

PWCs feel considerable gratitude toward the exceptional doctors who have respected us, believed in us, and treated us with compassion. Those doctors who practice the art as well as the science of medicine and who have devoted long hours to often-unpaid CFIDS research and treatment are truly special. We respect and appreciate them beyond measure.

UNPOPULAR TRUTHS

There is no magic bullet, no universally successful form of treatment. Any treatment carries the risk of potential harm; no one has all the answers; the doctor does not necessarily know best. Marcus Welby, M.D., is a fictional character; few if any medical professionals can offer the combination of knowledge, experience, warmth, and understanding that we crave. The bottom line is that we are responsible for our own medical decisions and care. We must educate ourselves, although our physicians may be less than thrilled if we are knowledgeable and curious.

We are not to blame when a treatment fails to help; most of the time no one is to blame. There is no target for our anger and frustration, and we must resist the temptation to appoint a scapegoat (the doctor, the medical profession, or ourselves).

Finding treatments and ultimately a cure for CFIDS is no simple matter. We would like to believe that there is a culprit (a germ, or something) that we can fight and eradicate. The true picture is more complex.

We may feel rejected by our doctors, often realistically so. They are the experts regarding medical practice; we are the experts regarding the functioning of our own bodies. A combination of these two levels of perception offers important information. Doctor and patient must work together as teammates. Doctors don't perform miracles, and medicine is not a perfect or exact science. The innate healing ability of our bodies is more magical than the "science" called medicine. Medical science offers a vast array of interventions that can facilitate healing, but *it is the body that heals*.

There is no such thing as "normal." What is typical of one person may be atypical for another. Normal represents an average, from which most people deviate to some degree. Each of us is unique and complex. We function differently and respond differently to treatment.

Seeking wellness is a trial-and-error process. Healing remains an art, a combination of scientific knowledge and the practitioner's skills. Our health care system is imperfect. Our task is to make use of its strengths but also to understand its weaknesses. Providers and consumers of health care together can create positive change in this system.

Chapter 11

◆

Treatment

W HEN DIAGNOSED WITH CFIDS, many of us asked, "Okay, so what do I take to make me better?" We were naive enough to believe that every illness had a cure. Our expectations changed as the grim reality set in: there is no specific, universally successful CFIDS treatment. We then began the search for treatments that would help us to feel better rather than get better. Finding a doctor willing to try alternatives, using educated guesswork, and medicating on a trial-and-error approach helped us to find the most beneficial treatments: a multifaceted treatment program that includes lifestyle modification most importantly, together with sleep improvement, avoidance of relapse triggers, and both general and symptomatic treatment.

Sara Reynolds, M.D., writes:

> We have an illness for which there is (1) no positive laboratory diagnosis (according to the recent CDC criteria) (2) no usual course, and (3) no specific treatment. Hence, there are many possibilities for untried remedies. There will be the uninformed or even unscrupulous who will suggest useless and/or very expensive, certainly unproved, remedies. There is a great temptation to feel that whatever you are taking when you begin to feel better must be the magic cure. (CFS *Jigsaw*, April 1988)

But because our symptoms wax and wane unpredictably, we cannot be sure that improvement is caused by medication. Dr. Reynolds suggests several trials, going on and off a particular medication until a definite correlation between it and symptom relief can be established.

Any treatment is potentially dangerous. The current trend toward the use of "natural" products is based upon the false assumption that "natural" equals "safe." Anything that enters the body can alter its functioning for better or for worse—or some of each. Mainstream doctors typically use pharma-ceutical drugs as a primary treatment modality, a good-news/bad-news proposition. Many medications ease suffering and save or prolong lives. However, medications can create new problems as they alleviate existing ones. Any substance powerful enough to affect body chemistry may cause serious side effects or severe complications. Many of today's "miracle" drugs will be deemed worthless or even harmful in the future. Thalidomide and DES are examples of pharmaceutical products once considered helpful and safe that later produced tragic results.

Also, little is really known about the complex interactions of various drugs taken simultaneously. This complicates things further. The results of treatment with pharmaceutical drugs can be magic or tragic—or somewhere in between. A fairly conservative yet open-minded approach to treatment makes the most sense.

When we feel awful, our concern about the risks of experimental treatment seem to decrease in inverse proportion to the severity of our symptoms. We try out various medications, weighing risk, fear, and uncertainty against the degree of desperation. We keep hope alive by continuing to try new things rather than waiting helplessly for the situation to resolve itself. We can't always know for certain what the long-term effects of a drug might be, but what is the alternative? Do we wait until a cure is discovered, refusing treatment in the interim? Do we wait for the results of scientifically valid, double-blind studies to ascertain the safety and effectiveness of a drug (which can take many years) and suffer in the meantime? As one patient said, "I'm spending all this money on drugs and medical care, and I'm just being experimented on, waiting for a cure."

Most of the available information about treatment results in PWCs is anecdotal, that is, based upon nonstandardized, informal clinical trials with differing numbers of patients—sometimes only a few. Anecdotal reports provide interesting leads as to what might be helpful. We need more systematic, scientific trials, which are expensive and time-consuming, but in the meantime we need symptom relief. Physicians are placed in a bind; they want to use medications wisely but cannot wait years for results of experimentation when their patients are ill _now_. Jay Goldstein, M.D., said at the 1987 CFS Convention in Oregon:

> I feel that when we are dealing with a disorder such as the chronic fatigue syndrome, you can't wait for double-blind experiments to tell you what to do. When I see a patient that has a problem for which there is no treatment anywhere in the medical literature, I feel that it is my responsibility and my obligation to use what I know as well as I can to help this person['s] suffering, even though it might be a treatment that no one has ever done before. I feel that it is a tragic failure of American medicine that they have lived in the straight jacket of the double-blind experiment. It's made doctors unnecessarily rigid, narrow, unthinking, and noncreative. That's what you don't need when you have a disease like [CFIDS].

Accepting that there is no standard treatment regimen for CFIDS is very difficult for doctor and patient. Deciding which treatments to try is confusing and frustrating. Evaluating the results of treatments is almost impossible, given the unpredictable course of CFIDS. Well-intentioned friends and family members offer advice and admonitions. ("There is a stigma now about taking drugs," said one patient. "It really bugs my mother and husband that I'm taking drugs. They think I shouldn't have to.") Our goal is to obtain as much help as possible while minimizing risks. As much as we would like to "just say no" to drugs, our need for relief is strong.

When a particular treatment seems to be effective, we are often told this is just a "placebo effect," as if the placebo response were synonymous with voodoo. It is actually the power of belief, the confidence in a treatment that can trigger us to

mobilize our own resources to obtain relief. Belief in the curative power of a treatment can be as potent as the treatment
itself; neither the mind (the patient's set of beliefs) nor the
body (the physiological effect of a treatment) can be considered
the sole source of a treatment's success; the interaction of the
two determines the result. Although a scientific rationale for a
treatment's apparent effectiveness is not always available, positive belief and hope are known to create physiological change.
Paul Cheney, M.D., views the placebo response as an expectation of wellness which causes the emission of polypeptides from
the central nervous system, improving immune function. He
believes that a positive attitude and active imagery have a
positive effect on the immune system (January 14, 1987). Other
physicians concur. "I try to get the patient to understand that
the *body* heals, not the therapy . . . . The most important thing
is to pick a therapy you believe in and proceed with a positive
attitude," writes Bernie Siegel, M.D., and Norman Cousins
describes the placebo as "the doctor who resides within."

Instilling hope in a PWC is one of the practitioner's most
valuable functions. On several occasions I saw my physician
during discouraging exacerbations, and his attitude alone
helped me to mobilize my will toward wellness before I even
began the new treatment. Knowing that there were still options
to try, that relief was possible, and that I had a good doctor on
my side kept me going.

I wrote in my journal:

> Sometimes I wonder what I should believe in. If I weren't so
> damned skeptical, something might have cured me already. If
> I could convince myself of the effectiveness of something, any-
> thing, I might get well . . . .
>
> Another new medicine, and the hope that maybe this will
> do it. I'd sell my soul for a magic pill. And then some weird-
> ass reaction to the medicine; there goes all the hope . . . until
> I hear about the next minor miracle, which I will doubtless
> try. I admire people who have total faith in something—reli-
> gion, herbs, whatever . . . . Hope is so important. Do I feel bet-
> ter because I get hopeful, or do I get hopeful when I'm feeling
> better? Both, I suspect.

Since then I have come to the realization that a belief system evolves—one does not simply self-impose an effective healing philosophy. Developing an understanding of the complex interactions between behavior, treatment options, and an emerging belief system is a process rather than an event.

When something—yoga, vitamins, pharmaceuticals, or acupuncture—seems to help, the properties of the treatment combined with the relief and sense of hope interact in a psychological-physiological process. Don't let anyone tell you that it's not "real," or that it's all in your head, or any other such nonsense. If you believe in it and it's helpful, the treatment is of value (as long as it does not have serious deleterious effects). If a treatment is effective initially but later loses its beneficial effects, it may be wise to discontinue it for a period of time and then restart it. If beneficial effects are not felt the second time around, eliminate the treatment and seek an alternative.

When a treatment seems to make the symptoms worse, we may be told that we are having a "healing crisis" and that our discomfort or pain results from "toxins" being expelled from our tissues. Although some medications cause initial side effects that do not persist, it is unclear whether a so-called healing crisis is a positive sign. If any form of treatment causes severe discomfort, seek competent medical advice immediately.

The spectrum of treatments undertaken by PWCs is amazingly diverse. Different physicians favor different treatment approaches, which are generally tailored to the needs of the individual and which may change over time as new discoveries are made. CFIDS practitioners have found that the results of treatment, even with the more promising drugs, are variable, producing significant alleviation of symptoms in some PWCs, moderate improvement in others, and no effects or an adverse effect in yet others.

One person's miracle treatment is another's poison. The success of some treatments may be short-term, and symptoms may return during a course of medication or after it is discontinued. The severity of the illness in individual cases determines how aggressive treatment should be.

Consult your doctor about treatment possibilities, and get information about options from CFIDS newsletters and journals. Consider the whole picture: not only the potential side effects of medications you are considering but also their possible interactions with other medications. Also consider the cost: many available treatments are not covered by medical insurance and you may want to check with your insurance carrier before initiating more expensive treatment. Because of a lack of scientific studies, all CFIDS treatments are considered experimental, and insurance companies are erratic and unpredictable in their reimbursement for CFIDS treatments.

Remember that drug combinations can be tricky. Make sure all physicians treating you have a list of all the medications you are taking, including over-the-counter remedies, vitamins and supplements, herbs, and birth control pills. Drug interactions can produce symptoms worse than the symptoms being treated by them and may even result in irreversible damage or death. Use of tobacco and/or alcohol can affect your response to medication and ideally both should be discontinued, or at least moderated.

CFIDS treatments are of two main types: primary treatment (aimed at treating the disease in general), and symptom-specific treatment. The following discussion of treatments is presented as general information rather than advice—treatment should be initiated *only under medical supervision.* In some cases the information is technical and may be of greater relevance to the practitioner than to the PWC. Because traditional dosages may not be appropriate for PWCs, practitioners should check with informed physicians or in the CFIDS literature, or call the CFIDS 800- or 900-numbers (see Appendix A) for current treatment information, including dosages.

(*Explanation of Abbreviations:* OTC indicates those treatments that are available over the counter [without a prescription]; IM indicates administration by intramuscular injection; IV indicates intravenous administration. The trade name of the medication is given first with the generic name in parentheses.)

PRIMARY THERAPY:
GENERAL TREATMENT OF CFIDS

Included in this category are treatments that have been reported to cause general improvement. Creating improved immune functioning and halting the action of viruses are important aspects of CFIDS treatment. Many of the medications are new and experimental, and most have antiviral or immune-modulating properties. In some, the mode of action is not well understood. Many of these medications are new and experimental. In using immunomodulating drugs, we face the "possibility of turning an unpleasant disease into a dangerous one" and need to examine possible serious side effects and long-term effects of subjecting an already-dysregulated immune system to these agents (Bell, 1991, p. 120).

Although the list of treatments is lengthy, the most effective and commonly used treatments currently include the tricyclic antidepressants (most commonly doxepin), Prozac, gamma globulin, H$_2$ blockers, and several newer medications. Others are listed either because they have been tried with good results or because they show promise and are currently being studied (e.g., Kutapressin, Ampligen, Ritanserin). Some medications that were originally considered promising but used with little success have been listed as well.

Adenosine monophosphate (AMP) is a natural cellular metabolite that has been used effectively for treatment of certain herpesviruses. AMP is believed to be most helpful in early stages of the illness. Clinicians report widely differing treatment results, but AMP has been quite helpful for some PWCs, who have reported general improvement, including decreased fatigue and increased energy. Side effects include asthma, shortness of breath and transient flushing, palpitation, and dizziness with high doses.

Alpha interferon (IFN), oral or injectable. Available only in its recombinant form as Roferon and Intron-A rather than its natural form, IFN is thought to have various immune-enhancing functions and may be more helpful in combination with other treatments than alone. Only small doses are used because of the poor risk/benefit ratio for high dosage use. Tests are currently underway using interferon for treatment of various viral conditions in humans. IFN should not be given if the patient already has detectable levels of alpha interferon.

AL721 (OTC): Active lipids in the ratio 7:2:1, a derivative of egg yolks which was developed in Israel. AL721 is available without a prescription through manufacturers and AIDS support/buying groups. It was initially believed to be produce overall improvement and is reported to be safe and free from side effects. However, it has not been very helpful in CFIDS treatment.

Ampligen is a biological response modulator with antiviral and immunomodulating properties that is currently being tested for use in CFIDS, AIDS, and cancer. Results of clinical trials with Ampligen have shown it to be a promising drug for CFIDS treatment. Improvements include better cognitive functioning (accompanied by an increase in IQ scores), increased activity levels and exercise tolerance, and decreased fatigue. It is believed to have few serious side effects (Peterson, Suhadolnik), but is quite expensive and is not yet FDA-approved.

Antibiotics are used to treat bacterial infections and are generally ineffective against viruses. Overuse and inappropriate use of antibiotics are major criticisms of allopathic medical practice today and are believed to play a part in encouraging candida (yeast) overgrowth. However, Vibramycin (doxycycline), a well-known antibiotic in the tetracycline class, has helped PWCs occasionally. No systematic CFIDS treatment studies of doxycycline have been conducted. It is generally safe, with such side effects as photosensitivity, candidiasis, and gastric complaints. It is most effective in children and those who have been ill short-term. The reason for its effectiveness is unknown; doxycycline may have immune-modulating properties.

Antifungals. Diflucan (fluconazole), Mycostatin (nystatin), and Nizoral (ketoconazole) are anti-candida/anti-fungal agents that may have overall positive effects in the treatment of CFIDS.

Further information is listed under "Symptomatic Treatment" below. New antifungals are being developed and are expected to be available in the near future.

Coenzyme Q10 (OTC) is thought to have immune-enhancing qualities and to affect ATP, the energy molecule in cells. Reports regarding the efficacy of CoQ10 are mixed and it is quite expensive. Large doses taken sublingually seem to be most effective, according to Paul Cheney, M.D. It is often used synergistically with other medications such as Prozac. Some patients report general improvement (increased energy level and improved muscle strength) after several weeks, but most seem to receive no benefit. CoQ10 is available at health food stores and from the CFIDS Buyers' Club (see Appendix A); prices vary widely for different brands.

DHEA is an adrenal steroid that may also be an immuno-modulator which affects metabolism. Some PWCs who have tried DHEA report symptom relief, but it is not widely used and may have a poor risk/benefit ratio.

Dimethylglycine (DMG) (OTC) is believed to be an immune modulator and metabolic enhancer. It has been used in combination with other immune boosters, but without remarkable results.

Gamma globulin is a blood product that contains antibodies. It is used especially when repeated upper respiratory infections occur and when total IgG is low and/or IgG subclass deficiencies exist. (IgG is one of several types of immunoglobins or antibodies which are produced in the lymph cells to combat foreign substances.) Although expensive and inconvenient (and in some cases not covered by medical insurance), IV administration of gamma globulin is usually more effective than IM administration. Jay Goldstein, M.D., advises measuring IgA levels and anti-IgA antibodies before gamma globulin is given to avoid serum sickness. Treatment may need to be aggressive (high doses at frequent intervals) in order to be effective. Some PWCs may have an allergic reaction to gamma globulin and some may have an excitatory response, which is atypical of the general population. Other side effects at high doses include phlebitis, headache, nausea, malaise, and transiently abnormal liver function tests. Results of experimental trials are inconsistent; some resulted in improvement in about half of those treated, others showed little or no benefit. Dosages vary widely. High-dose administration is likely to cause side effects, but if the dosage is too low no benefit will be realized. Those who experience greatest benefit initially may find this treatment losing its effect over time.

Germanium (in the form of germanium sesquioxide) (OTC) has been used to treat chronic viral infection and other disorders. In other than the sesquioxide form, germanium can cause severe side effects, including renal (kidney) failure. Germanium is not generally considered effective in treating CFIDS, but its proponents claim that those who have tried it have taken doses that are too low to be effective and may have taken a poor quality product.

H2 blockers such as Zantac (ranitidine), Tagamet (cimetidine), Pepcid (famotidine), and Axid (nizatidine) are generally prescribed for gastric complaints (they suppress production of stomach acids) but seem to have general beneficial results for some PWCs. If one of the H2 blockers proves ineffective, another may be successful; some PWCs respond to one but not to the others. Insomnia and agitation are unusual side effects in the general population but are experienced by some PWCs, so it is wise to start with a small dose and increase gradually (Gold-stein). Some patients are helped significantly (usually after several days or weeks), some are helped somewhat, and about 50% report no benefit.

Hydrogen peroxide (food grade only; OTC) in a highly diluted form and other hyperoxygenation agents (hyperbaric oxygen, ozone therapy, hypochlorous acid) are reported to have helped some PWCs but have not generally had an impressive record. Additionally, the poor risk-benefit ratio and lack of scientific rationale have led most practitioners to avoid this type of treatment.

Inosine pranobex (Isoprinosine or Pranocin; OTC in some countries), thought to be an immune enhancer, has not received FDA approval and is unavailable in the United States. It is manufactured and sold in many countries, including Mexico. Inosine pranobex is used to treat illnesses characterized by immune deficiencies and has received mixed reviews from PWCs. The optimum dose is unknown, as is the method of action. Side effects are rare; some patients experience mild nausea and/or a transient rise in serum and urinary uric acid levels. Only preliminary studies have been conducted thus far, with contradictory results.

Kutapressin is a liver derivative complex (a mixture of peptides and amino acids) that may serve as an immuno-modulator or antiviral agent. It may have a beneficial effect on CFIDS patients when given by injection. It is FDA-approved and has been used to treat such disorders as neurasthenia, skin problems, and shingles. There are no known side effects, other than local skin reactions when given by injection. Informal testing with CFIDS patients has produced good general results; further studies are being conducted. Kutapressin may improve fatigue and endurance, help herpes blisters and shingles, and sometimes reduce pain. It does not help cognitive impairment, however. Kutapressin may be used in combination with other therapies.

L-Carnitine (OTC) may be used for cardiac irregularities, muscle weakness, and low body temperature, but has caused weight gain in some patients.

Lentinus edodes mycelium, LEM, a Shiitake mushroom extract (OTC) is believed to improve immune functioning and has been used in the treatment of AIDS. It has been widely used in Japan; studies are currently being conducted in the United States. LEM is expensive and generally not covered by medical insurance. Reported effective by about half of those who have tried it, LEM loses its benefits over time in some cases. It is believed to increase the number of white blood cells, especially NK cells. Letinan is an extract from another part of the same mushroom which differs somewhat from LEM, although both are believed to have antiviral properties.

L-lysine (OTC) is an amino acid that is inexpensive and readily available. It is used to control herpes simplex lesions, including mouth ulcers and cold sores. Lysine may be most effective when combined with a low-arginine diet (another amino acid found in such foods as chocolate, carob, whole grains, raisins, nuts, and seeds). It is thought to be nontoxic even in large doses.

Monolauren (OTC) is a patented monoglyceride ester of lauric acid (a fatty acid), which may be effective against lipid-enveloped viruses (herpesviruses and others) by inhibiting virus cells from attaching to host cells, thereby halting viral replication. Monolauren is believed to be nontoxic, but has not proven very effective in the treatment of CFIDS and is not widely used.

Naltrexone (Trexan) is commonly used in treatment of drug addictions. In CFIDS treatment it has been used alone or in combination with other drugs to boost natural killer cell activity and possibly improve cognitive functioning and sleep (decrease nightmares and "sleep seizures"). Clinicians have reported mixed results; many patients react adversely even to low doses. When improvement does occur, it takes about a month.

Omega-6 free fatty acids (Evening Primrose Oil) and **omega-3 fatty acids** (EPA Fish Oil) (OTC) affect the prostaglandins (mediators of pain and inflammation) and the cyto-kines. They may be helpful for pain when combined with antiinflammatory drugs, including aspirin and ibuprofen. Most anecdotal reports indicate no significant benefit, but at least one preliminary study has shown improvement in some PWCs who use essential fatty acids.

Prozac (fluoxetine) is a relatively new antidepressant that increases the amount of serotonin available at the neural synapses (in the brain) and may have immunomodulating properties. Prozac is relatively expensive and tends to energize patients, at least initially. Although Prozac often relieves multiple CFIDS symptoms, it does not improve sleep; conversely, it may cause insomnia and increased anxiety in certain individuals. It is extremely helpful in reducing mood swings, usually within a few days, and may decrease pain and cause overall improvement. Side effects include rash and gastrointestinal upset, anxiety, decrease in sexual interest, and delayed orgasm. Recent claims of the dangers of Prozac—warning of out-of-control episodes resulting in homicides and suicides—have been invalidated. However, Prozac is not a harmless drug and should be prescribed with caution. PWCs may not tolerate high doses and usually start with small amounts, increasing as necessary. Wellbutrin (bupropion) may be effective if Prozac is ineffective or not well tolerated.

Retrovir (zidovudine; AZT) is an antiviral used for treating retrovirus-related illness. Although AZT is FDA-approved and widely used to treat HIV disease, its application in CFIDS treatment is unknown and untested at present. AZT is quite expensive and not well tolerated by many patients. It is not recommended for CFIDS treatment except for PWCs who are HIV positive and have low T4 counts.

Ribavirin is an antiviral that has been used in the treatment of AIDS. Its potential side effects (bone marrow problems, suppression of white blood cells) make it a poor choice for CFIDS treatment. It may have some value in treatment of viral/immune problems, but its safety is questionable and it has not been used or recommended often in the treatment of CFIDS. It is expensive and difficult to obtain.

Ritanserin is a long-acting 5-HT2 receptor blocker that has antidepressant and antianxiety properties. Preliminary reports of Dr. Jay Goldstein's study show improved sleep and decreased pain and daytime fatigue among a small number of PWCs, who showed great variance in their responsiveness to the drug, although all tolerated it well. In those who were helped, symptoms quickly returned when the drug was discontinued. Further studies are expected.

Thymic hormone has been investigated by Nathan Trainin, M.D., of the Weizmann Institute in Israel. Thymic humoral factor (THF) may enhance the production of T-lymphocytes and may prove helpful in viral treatment, but it remains an unknown in CFIDS treatment.

Transfer factor (TF) is a blood product containing cells from the blood of an individual who is intimate with the PWC but not ill (for example, a spouse or other household member). The blood is processed according to an elaborate procedure, and TF is administered by injection. Results have been spotty; although some practitioners claim great success with transfer factor, most have not found it effective. Its use is considered highly experimental, and Jay Goldstein, M.D., recommends it only as a last resort.

Tricyclic antidepressants: Sinequan or Adapin (doxepin) is a tricyclic antidepressant that may have immunomodulating properties. It improves sleep and reduces pain for many PWCs and is a commonly used and effective treatment. Doxepin has also helped with these symptoms: nasal allergies, gastritis, fever, functional level, general fatigue, and neurological symptoms. Although other antidepressants have been beneficial—those in both the tricyclic and monamine oxidase inhibitor (MAOI) classes—doxepin is most widely used in treating CFIDS. If doxepin is not well tolerated, Pamelor (which is less sedating) or other tricyclics may be tried. Doxepin and other tricyclics may cause side effects, including dry mouth, constipation, and weight gain.

Vitamin-mineral supplements (most OTC): These should preferably be good quality, yeast- and sugar-free, high in the B vitamins as well as vitamins C, A and E, and containing minerals —especially zinc, potassium, and magnesium. Such supplementation is important for PWCs because vitamins and minerals may be depleted or poorly absorbed. Those suggested by various physicians include Berocca Plus (by prescription), or Optivite, MaxiLife, Theragran M, Centrum, or Stresstab, which are available OTC. Additional supplements such as vitamins C and B-12 are recommended and are discussed separately.

Vitamin B-12 (oral OTC, nasal gel, or injectable by prescription) has helped some CFIDS patients, even when blood levels of B-12 are normal. B-12 may provide an energy boost and may help with neurological and overall symptoms. When taking high doses of B-12 it is wise to take a multivitamin or B-complex supplement which will supply large amounts of the other B vitamins. The effectiveness of B-12 may wear off; if so it may be discontinued and restarted a few weeks later.

Vitamin C (oral or IV, tablets available OTC) is thought to produce hyperoxygenation/free radical increase and may have other beneficial effects as well. The use of high-dose intravenous vitamin C is considered controversial; some practitioners report dramatic positive results and others find such treatment ineffective and even potentially dangerous. Taken orally, vitamin C may produce gastric complaints; if so, the dosage should be lowered and increased gradually.

Zovirax (acyclovir) is used orally or IV to combat multiple herpes group viruses. Once believed to be a promising CFIDS treatment, Zovirax has been found to be occasionally helpful and is often tried when viral involvement has been shown and other treatments have not been successful. Symptoms generally return when it is discontinued and its long-term effects are unknown. Acyclovir has application in certain viral disorders, but further systematic testing is needed to determine its appropriate use and dosage. Zovirax is quite expensive.

NUTRITION, SUPPLEMENTS, AND ENVIRONMENTAL TOXINS

I can resist everything except temptation.
Oscar Wilde

Ours is a nutrition-conscious age in which "natural" products are widely advertised and self-proclaimed nutrition experts abound. Health stores and bookstores offer a wealth of information and misinformation about nutritional programs and products, often loaded with contradictory and inflated claims.

Medical schools have typically paid little attention to nutrition, yet we often turn to our physicians for nutritional advice. Fortunately many medical schools are now requiring courses in nutrition and research in this area is flourishing.

As we become aware of the effects of pollution on our environment, we worry about contaminated water, or foods grown in depleted soil and loaded with pesticides and antibiotics. We are bombarded with media-borne proclamations that we need fiber, complex carbohydrates, lean meat or none at all, fresh veggies . . . and yet our convenience stores and restaurants carry few or none of these products. We become suspicious that any food we enjoy is likely to contribute to an early demise. And when we develop CFIDS, one "expert" tells us to load up on protein; another tells us to eat small amounts. One expert tells us to eat a diet high in complex carbohydrates, another tells us that all carbohydrates can contribute to yeast overgrowth. When energy is low, we may crave sugar and carbohydrates ("junk food syndrome")—the very things we know must be bad for us. What to do? Who's right? There are no simple answers.

Vitamins and minerals Certain vitamins seem to enhance well-being and healthy immune functioning, but we don't really know what they do outside the laboratory, inside the body. We should not assume that vitamins and other nutritional supplements are harmless: anything taken in large enough doses can be toxic, and some substances (including "natural" ones) are harmful even in small amounts. Nor should we rely on self-proclaimed noncredentialed "health experts," such as the clerks in health food stores whose job is to sell you their products (often whatever is overstocked or a fad "wonder" product touted in a nonscientific publication). Consult a well-trained nutritionist before embarking on a program of supplementation.

In addition to the vitamins, minerals, and supplements listed above, the following have been suggested by various physicians who treat CFIDS: zinc, niacinamide, folic acid, vitamin E, selenium, lecithin, calcium, beta-carotene, certain amino acids, and various commercially-produced "immune boosting" preparations. Certain extracts (adrenal, thymus, and pancreatic) have been mentioned as treatment options by some practitioners but are regarded with skepticism by others. Finally, "metabolic clearing therapy" is a detox program in which "assault chemicals" from the environment are cleared from the body, allowing the immune system to function more productively. The program consists of protein, vitamin, mineral, and enzyme products loaded with antioxidants, to which certain foods are gradually added as observations for food allergies are made. I know of no scientific studies regarding the success of these programs.

Herbal remedies Herbs have been used for centuries to treat various illnesses. Unfortunately the scientific study of herbal remedies is not advanced, and the benefits and dangers associated with them are often unknown. Chinese herbs and other herbal remedies have reportedly helped some patients, while adverse effects of certain herbal preparations have also been reported, including worsening of CFIDS symptoms and allergic reactions. Some substances that are not FDA-approved and available only in other countries may contain steroids, which produce a sense of well-being but may cause long-term problems (Sara Reynolds, M.D.).

Herbal regimens offered by Sunrider and other manufacturers offer promises of symptom improvement and enhancement of the body's total balance and healing ability—but not a cure. Such herbal preparations include Dong Quai (analgesic, muscle-relaxant, antiallergenic); ginseng (central nervous system stimulant, improves circulation, improves glandular functioning); Ma Huang (antiallergy and asthma, weight loss), Fo-Ti (sedative, anti-tumor, blood fortification); and Ginkgo Biloba (improved cognitive/neurological functioning); astragalus; echinacea; garlic; and milk thistle (for liver involvement). Herbs are generally used synergystically and should be taken under the supervision of an expert with proper training and experience. One drawback is the expense of many such herbal programs. Many PWCs have had excellent responses to herbal treatment but others have not. "These kinds of revelations

should be viewed with both hope and caution," wrote Marc M.
Iverson in *The CFIDS Chronicle* (January/February 1989, p. 51).
Lack of scientific studies and consistent results make all claims
of effectiveness provisional. Because good results have been
obtained in some cases, the use of herbs warrants further study.

Diet. General diet suggestions for PWCs include:

> the judicious use of certain vitamins and supplements
> a diet high in vegetables and complex carbohydrates
>   and moderate in protein
> a diet low in fats (especially saturated fats), sodium, and
>   processed foods
> avoidance of caffeine, alcohol, nicotine, sugars, and
>   other refined carbohydrates, including white flour
> fresh foods rather than canned, frozen, or processed ones
> small, frequent meals

Individual experimentation is the most accurate method
of determining which foods are well-tolerated and which ones
are not. PWCs may be sensitive to food additives, dyes, and
antibiotics; dairy products; gluten products; aspartame; MSG;
certain spices; sulfites; nitrates; some hard-to-digest vegetables.
An elimination diet combined with careful record-keeping
under medical supervision may help to uncover food allergies
and sensitivities. Symptoms of food intolerance include malaise,
mood alteration, digestive disturbances, food cravings, and
repetitive eating patterns. Skin and blood tests are generally
considered unreliable in diagnosing food allergies.

Some PWCs report carbohydrate cravings, especially during exacerbations. Although a psychological basis for these
cravings has been suggested, there is evidence that the source
is largely physiological, possibly a chemical problem related to
levels of serotonin and/or other neurotransmitters or to systemic yeast infection. Consumption of simple carbohydrates
may increase fatigue, causing a "boost-and-crash" cycle (as the
blood sugar level rises and then plummets quickly and dramatically) and perhaps compounding candida-related problems and

other symptoms. The problem can be dealt with by limiting the consumption of simple carbohydrates. Complex carbohydrates are metabolized more slowly and don't cause the "boost and crash" effect.

Avoiding environmental toxins. Many CFIDS patients are especially sensitive to environmental pollutants and chemicals. Immune suppression is thought to be related to the immune system's difficulty in coping with numerous substances with which we come into contact. Avoidance of all toxic substances is not possible, but we need to exercise caution whenever possible to minimize adding to the total body load, which adversely affects our already-compromised immune systems. Many CFIDS patients find they are sensitive to some or all of the following: hairsprays, perfumes, pesticides, chemicals, cleaning products, fuels and exhaust fumes, and tung oil (found in varnish, shellac, and some furniture oils and paint products).

SYMPTOMATIC TREATMENT

Anxiety

In addition to general relaxation techniques, which must be practiced regularly in order to be effective, minor tranquilizers are helpful. Those most commonly prescribed are Xanax (alprazolam), BuSpar (buspirone), and Valium (diazepam), although Klonopin (clonazepam) may also be helpful in treating anxiety disorders. Valium is no longer generally used because it can cause depression as a side effect and may be addictive. Xanax is a popularly prescribed medication that alleviates anxiety and seems to have antidepressant properties as well. Because it produces drowsiness, many PWCs with sleep disorders use Xanax to help them to fall asleep. It may be addictive, however, and sudden withdrawal is accompanied by withdrawal symptoms. BuSpar is an antianxiety agent that is not related to the benzodiazepines; it is nonaddictive and does not cause the same severe withdrawal effects as Valium and Xanax. BuSpar does not cause sedation or the mild sense of euphoria associated with

Xanax and Valium, and may be used along with Klonopin, which is sedating.

For the treatment of occasional anxiety these medications can be taken as needed. For more constant generalized anxiety, daily medication is appropriate. The tricyclic antidepressant Imipramine is helpful for panic disorder and should be taken on a regular basis to be effective.

Cognitive dysfunction

The following medications have been used to treat cognitive dysfunction:

Calan SR (verapamil HCl)

Calcium channel blockers, e.g., Nimotop (nimodipine), Hydergine (ergoloid mesylates), Cardene (nicardipine HCl), Procardia (nifedipine), have been used with varying resul

Diamox (acetazolamide)

Dynagen

Ionamin (phentermine), Cylert (pemoline) or Ritalin (methylphenidate)

Nootrapil (Piracetam): not yet available in the U.S.

Symmetrel (amantadine HCl) should be avoided in those with a history of seizures or congestive heart failure; may be discontinued and restarted if it loses its effectiveness

Tegretol (carbamaxzepine), Depakene (valproic acid), Depakote (divalproex sodium), and Klonopin (clonazepam): especially useful when there is temporal lobe involvement; may also help anxiety and panic disorder as well as seizure-like episodes

Trexan (naltrexone): specially diluted in small doses (should be avoided if narcotic analgesics are frequently used)

Vasopressin: desmopressin acetate (DDAVP)

(Cheney, Goldstein, Rubin)

Some of the above medications, e.g., calcium channel blockers, must be taken for several weeks before effects will be felt. Medications for other symptoms, e.g., Prozac, Seldane, and vitamin B-12 along with Coenzyme Q10, improve cognition in some cases.

Cognitive retraining, provided by certain neuropsychologists and neuropsychiatrists, is instructive for those with cognitive dysfunction, including memory problems. Linda Miller Iger, Ph.D., Tarras Onischenko, Ph.D., and Curt Sandman, Ph.D., have worked extensively with PWCs experiencing cognitive dysfunction and have developed a series of techniques for enhancing memory and cognition. A special issue of _The CFIDS Chronicle_ (August 1991) focused exclusively on their work. Some of the tools and techniques are used by psychologists specializing in cognitive restructuring and by specially trained occupational therapists; others may be implemented individually by the PWC and a companion.

Depression

Antidepressants, most commonly those in the tricyclic class, are commonly used in the treatment of CFIDS. The tricyclics treat depression by affecting brain chemicals. As added benefits, certain antidepressants function as antihistamines and anti-inflammatories, helping with sleep disorders and pain. They are nonaddictive and should be taken regularly rather than sporadically to obtain full benefit. Common side effects of tricyclics include anticholinergic effects: dry mouth, constipation, and weight gain. Because many CFIDS patients are exquisitely sensitive to medications, dosages should be started at extremely low levels and increased to the individual's optimal dose. Doxepin is considered the most helpful of the tricyclics, although others in this class such as Pamelor (nortriptyline) and Tofranil (imipra-mine) have been helpful as well. Most often, a patient is started on small doses of doxepin, which are increased gradually if the drug is well tolerated. If not, other tricyclics may be tried until an effective one without significant deleterious side effects is found. Tricyclic antidepressants are among the very few CFIDS treatments almost universally endorsed among the experts! Tricyclic antidepressants do not provide a cure but offer significant relief of specific symptoms (especially depression and sleep disorders) and increased feelings of well-being for many. Low-dose thyroid medication is often administered along with antidepressants to enhance their effects.

Monamine oxidase inhibitors (MAOIs), another group of antidepressants, have also been used with success in treating CFIDS symptoms. Because of potential side effects and the dietary restrictions necessitated by MAOIs, they are often used only when treatment with tricyclics is unsuccessful. Parnate (tranylcypromine sulfate) and Nardil (phenelzine sulfate) seem to have immunologic effects. Irena Brus, M.D., a private practitioner and professor of clinical medicine at Mount Sinai School of Medicine in New York, found Nardil to be an effective CFIDS treatment, unfortunately with significant side effects, which caused some PWCs to discontinue the medication.

Lithium, a drug used to treat bipolar mood disorder (manic-depressive syndrome), has not shown promise in CFIDS treatment.

Prozac (fluoxetine HCl), described earlier, is a very effective antidepressant that causes improvement of other CFIDS symptoms, notably mood swings and sometimes energy level. Some PWCs report an initial "high"—a temporary energy boost often accompanied by weight loss. Prozac is long-acting, and its full effects may not be present until about four weeks after treatment is begun. Simultaneous treatment with Prozac and BuSpar may increase benefits.

Wellbutrin (bupropion) is a new antidepressant that does not cause the side effects commonly found in the tricyclics and MAOIs. Many PWCs report successful treatment with Wellbutrin, but an occasional side effect of Wellbutrin is seizures in a minority of patients with a predisposition to or a family history of seizure disorder. If an individual's depression is unresponsive to usual doses of these medications, an orthomolecular psychiatrist who specializes in the use of various combinations of drugs should be consulted.

Digestive problems

Sara Reynolds, M.D., wrote a helpful column on the treatment of digestive disorders in the August 1988 Phoenix CFS newsletter:

> Heartburn or reflux of stomach acid can be helped with antacids, avoidance of alcohol and spicy foods, and not eating within 3 to 4 hours of bedtime. Tagamet, Zantac, or other H_2 blockers available by prescription decrease the production of stomach acid.
>
> Metamucil, Kaopectate, Donnagel, Pepto-Bismol, and other OTC preparations may help control diarrhea. Adequate fluids should be taken in; bananas and applesauce may be helpful. If these remedies are ineffective, prescription medication (such as Lomotil) should be obtained from your physician.
>
> Stool softeners and bulk laxatives, as well as a diet high in liquids and fiber, including fresh fruits and vegetables, can ease constipation, as can exercise (if possible).
>
> For gas, indigestion and nausea, OTC preparations such as antacids, Alka-Seltzer, and Pepto-Bismol may help, as may dietary adjustments such as decreased intake of alcohol, caffeine, simple sugars and fats, and the elimination of nicotine.

Such medications as Tigan, Phenergan (promethazine), Peri-actin (cyproheptadine HCl), Ativan (lorazepam), and Antivert (meclizine HCl) may be helpful for the treatment of nausea. Antispasmodics such as Librax, Bentyl, Donnatal, and Isordil relieve spasms of smooth muscles, such as those in the intestinal tract. Patients have reported beneficial effects of PCD, a digestive aid, and charcoal tablets to reduce gas and bloating. The following medications have also been helpful with irritable bowel syndrome-type symptoms: Klonopin, calcium channel blockers, tricyclic antidepressants, Imodium (loperamide HCl) and, in severe treatment-resistant cases, Lupron (leuprolide ace-tate). Intestinal bloating and other symptoms may be relieved by anti-fungal (anti-candida) medication.

Food sensitivities/allergies and giardia or other intestinal parasites may be the cause of persistent symptoms and should be investigated if symptoms are severe and persistent.

Edema (swelling)

Edema, or swelling due to fluid retention, may be reduced by the use of diuretics. Extended use of diuretics for this purpose is not advised and many doctors do not even prescribe diuretics even for short-term use.

Cutting down on sodium intake (not only salt added in cooking or at the table, but sodium found in prepared foods), exercising if advisable, and increasing fluid intake are nondrug approaches to the problem of fluid retention.

Endometriosis

Endometriosis seems to affect PWCs in higher percentages than the general population, for reasons that are not understood. Treatments include medications such as progestational agents, and surgery in severe cases.

Energy improvement

Various general treatments discussed earlier may be helpful for boosting energy according to many physicians, including Drs. Cheney and Goldstein.

> Alpha interferon (low dose)
> Oral acyclovir (high dose)
> Doxycycline or low-dose tetracycline
> Kutapressin
> Vitamin B-12, alone or in combination with Coenzyme
>   Q10, preferably sublingually
> Vitamin B-6 (taken with other B vitamins)
> Adenosine monophosphate
> Naltrexone (a low-dose syrup may be specifically
>   prepared by physicians or pharmacists)

Antidepressants (Prozac)
MAOIs, especially Parnate
Wellbutrin
Deprenyl (a new MAOI-B inhibitor)
Symmetrel (amantadine) for flu-like symptoms
Acupuncture, acupressure

Fever

Anti-inflammatory medicines such as aspirin, ibuprofen, and acetaminophen are often used to bring down fevers. Some doctors caution against this practice except with extremely high fevers, since an elevated temperature is one of the body's natural ways of fighting infection. In fact, a slightly elevated body temperature may be detrimental to viral reproduction and thus be beneficial to the patient.

Headache

In a column called "The Excruciating Headache," Alan S. Goldberg described "my brain having a vendetta with my cranium." His remedy is the "deep freeze": he stores bags of antifreeze in his freezer and applies them to his head and the back of his neck in a darkened room. Although the cold is uncomfortable, he often obtains relief within a few minutes (*The CFIDS Chronicle,* April 1988, p. 19). Similar relief may be obtained by using "blue ice" packs or specially-designed facial masks that can be chilled.

Aspirin, acetaminophen (Tylenol and generics), and ibuprofen (Advil or other brands) may help headaches; stronger medications are indicated for more severe headaches. The treatment of allergic rhinitis often leads to improvement of other symptoms, including headache (Mease).

Paul Cheney, M.D. makes the following recommendations:

Pressure-like headaches:
— Diamox LA (acetazolamide)

Migraine-like headaches:
— high-dose long-acting calcium channel blockers such
  as Calan-SR (verapamil HCl) or Procardia-SR
  (nifedipine)
— If severe or acute: Nubaine (nalpuphine HCl) with
  Phenergan (promethazine HCl); Vicodin
  (hydrocodone bitartrate + acetaminophen); Darvocet
  (pro-posyphene napsylate + acetaminophen); Tylenol
  (acetaminophen) with codeine

Muscle tension headaches:
— Relaxation techniques
— TENS unit
— pressure point therapy
— Omega-3 or -6 and/or Advil or other
  anti-inflammatories

Nonspecific head pain:
— Tegretol (carbamazepine)
— treatment of sinus problems
— low-dose Xanax or Klonopin

(*The Mass. CFIDS Update*, Winter 1990)

Midrin (isometheptene mucate, dichloralphenazone + acetaminophen) may be helpful, as may Demerol (meperidine) in
the case of severe headaches that do not respond to other
medications.

Nasal congestion and sinus pain

Nasal congestion, sinus problems, and allergies are common
complaints among PWCs. Many report increased allergic symptoms that are not relieved by allergy injections. Antihistamines
are available OTC and by prescription. Most cause drowsiness
but certain newer prescription antihistamines such as Seldane
(terfenadine) and Hismanal (astemizole) do not.

Decongestants, available OTC or by prescription, reduce
nasal and sinus congestion. They may cause a feeling of being

"wired" and may interfere with sleep. Sometimes a combination decongestant/antihistamine is the most effective approach, and minimal dosages (even pediatric doses) may be useful if one is particularly sensitive. Often antibiotics, decongestants, steroid inhalers, and Nasalcrom (cromolyn sodium nasal solution) inhalers may also be helpful.

Joint and muscle pain

Body aches may be relieved with aspirin, acetaminophen, or ibuprofen (OTC). When sleep problems are successfully treated, pain may improve as a result. For more severe and persistent body aches stronger medications are generally used:

> Sinequan, used alone or synergistically with pain medications
> Captopril
> Tegretol (carbamazepine)
> Anti-inflammatories such as Naprosyn (naproxen) and Feldene (piroxicam) for arthritis-like pain
> Muscle relaxants such as Robaxin (methocarbamol), Parafon Forte (chlorzoxazone), Flexeril (cyclobenzaprine), and Norflex (orphenadrine) for muscle pain
> Soma (carisoprodol)
> Sandostatin (octreotide acetate) by injection
> Toradol, an anti-inflammatory drug, may relieve severe chronic pain.

Jay Goldstein, M.D., reports pain relief with low-dose naltrexone and with angiotensin-converting enzyme inhibitors, especially Vasotec (enalaprilat). Low doses of Klonopin or Xanax may also be helpful, as may be different combinations of drugs, for example, Xanax and ibuprofen, or doxepin and naproxen.

Many pain medications produce drowsiness as a side effect. Steroids (cortisone, prednisone, and ACTH—which increases production of steroids) are not recommended because of serious long-term side effects. Narcotic pain relievers should only be used on a short-term basis; long-term use may lead to acceleration of pain and addiction.

A comprehensive approach to the management of severe, continuing pain often includes biofeedback, passive stretching exercises, audiotaped relaxation/stress reduction exercises (see Chapter 14), trigger point therapy, myotherapy, tender point injections with saline or local anesthetics, and massage. Warm baths or sitting in a hot tub can bring pain relief. For pain in the legs and backs of the knees, lying with a pillow under the knees is helpful. Pain management clinics usually offer a multidisciplinary approach that includes biofeedback, relaxation training, physical therapy, and psychotherapy.

Sleep disorders

Treating the sleep disorders associated with CFIDS is very important. Improving sleep often leads to general symptom alleviation. Low-dose doxepin is often helpful. Although doxepin is preferred for its sleep-enhancing and other beneficial properties, other tricyclic antidepressants are helpful in sleep restoration, e.g., Triavil (perphenazine + amytriptilene 2-25), Desyrel and Pamelor. Drug choice should be based on individual symptoms and reactions to medication. OTC sleep-inducing medications include Benadryl, also available generically as diphenhydramine hydrochloride, and Unisom (doxylamine succinate). Prescription sleeping medications, such as Halcion or Restoril, can be helpful but are not advisable for long-term use. Low-dose Klonopin (clonazepam) improves the quality of sleep; side effects are not usually experienced. Since it is habituating, Klonopin should be discontinued periodically, it is generally tapered gradually over a period of thirty days when discontinued. Klonopin and Sinequan are often used synergistically to promote sleep. Low-dose Xanax may be helpful; its addicting properties should prompt one to exercise caution with high-doses or long-term use.

L-tryptophan is an amino acid that had served as a sleep-promoting agent. However, its sale has been banned because of serious complications found in some individuals using the product, and it should not be used.

Techniques for improving sleep suggested by Dr. Harvey Moldofsky at the Los Angeles CFS/FM Symposium include: maintaining a regular sleep schedule; determining the optimum number of hours of sleep needed; improving the sleeping environment (e.g., eliminating noise); exercising if appropriate; avoiding caffeine, alcohol, and tobacco; and avoiding naps if they interfere with regular sleep. Many PWCs find relaxation tapes and self-hypnosis helpful.

Urinary tract symptoms

In *You Don't Have to Live with Cystitis!*, Larrian Gillespie, M.D., recommends treatment suggestions, including medication and diet, for interstitial cystitis, a fairly common problem among PWCs, primarily women. She cautions against routine use of antibiotics for bladder problems, stating that antibiotic use is indicated only when a urine culture shows the presence of bacterial infection.

Minipress (prazosin HCl) is often helpful in the treatment of urinary tract problems, especially prostate problems in men.

Vestibular (balance) disorders

Medications helpful in treating balance disorders include:

motion sickness medications (e.g., dramamine, meclizine, scopolamine)
various B-vitamin preparations (orally or by injection)
antihistamines
stimulants (e.g., Cylert, Ritalin)
tranquilizers, antidepressants (used as "secondary" medications to treat persistent anxiety which often accompanies vestibular disorders)

(Reynolds, *CFS Bulletin*, May 1988; Levinson, 1986)

Lifestyle modification, diet, and surgery are other treatments used for various types of balance disorders. In his book *Phobia Free*, Harold Levinson discusses the connections between anxiety, phobias, certain learning disabilities, and inner ear disorders. His book contains suggestions regarding specific medications.

In their book *Balancing Act*, Mary Ann Watson, M.A., and Helen Sinclair, R.N., M.S., offer many suggestions, including:

> For acute vertigo: immobilize the head; fix the eyes on something stable; don't move until the nausea subsides and then do so gradually
>
> Minimize stress
>
> Explain your limitations to your family
>
> Drink adequate fluids; avoid alcohol; limit sodium, caffeine, and sugar
>
> Exercise if possible
>
> Avoid fatigue
>
> Take safety precautions to avoid injury

Try to become aware of triggers of balance problems (e.g., competing sensory input, fluorescent lights, bright lights, certain foods, activities, or body movements), and avoid or minimize them.

Some doctors attribute the "spacey feeling" (as opposed to dizziness or vertigo) to candidiasis and report that their patients are helped by an anticandida diet and medication.

If you are seeking treatment for a vestibular disorder and your family practitioner has not been able to help, ask for a referral to an otorhinolaryngologist or neuro-otologist.

Weight gain

Several nonamphetamine appetite-suppressant prescription medicines are available but are often not recommended by medical practitioners. These are intended only for short-term use and have some undesirable side effects, including a "wired" feeling that may interfere with sleep. The efficacy of such medications may be short-lived. Crash dieting and strenuous exercise are strongly discouraged for PWCs, who are likely to become sicker on such programs. Because certain medications can cause weight gain, it is wise to become familiar with the literature on all medications and supplements being used.

Thyroid tests are often performed, including one for anti-thyroid antibodies. Various thyroid supplements have been pre-scribed for PWCs: Synthroid, Armour thyroid, and Cytomel (liothyronine sodium). Considerable debate continues regard-ing the use of thyroid medication when thyroid tests are within the normal range, and whether thyroid supplements are ap-propriate in the treatment of CFIDS. Thyroid medication is not a miracle weight-loss drug and should not be used unless indi-cated.

DHEA, a steroid secreted by the adrenal cortex, may be low in some PWCs and is claimed to be an anti-obesity, anti-AIDS, anti-aging, and anti-stress hormone. It may be helpful in the treatment of PWCs who have gained fifty pounds or more. The risk/benefit ratio of DHEA is questionable and it is not available in the United States. When we are better able to understand the reason for the CFIDS-related weight gain in the absence of dietary change we may find new solutions to this problem.

Yeast/fungal overgrowth: candidiasis

The phenomenon of generalized yeast infections or overgrowth of _candida albicans_ is a controversial issue. Some doctors believe that most CFIDS patients have this problem and others believe that the condition is rare or nonexistent. Existing laboratory tests for candidiasis are expensive and unreliable, and there are no clear diagnostic criteria. Much of the literature about can-didiasis and treatment approaches is anecdotal and unscientific, and is therefore regarded with skepticism by the medical com-munity.

Symptoms of candidiasis include bloating, gas, diarrhea, and other digestive problems; mental "spaceyness"; rectal and/or vaginal irritation and itching; white-coated tongue ("thrush"); carbohydrate cravings; and skin and nail problems. Some of the popular books about candidiasis list almost every symptom in the world as being related to yeast infection, including most of the CFIDS symptoms we experience. It is unclear whether there is a causal connection between CFIDS and candidiasis or whether a weakened immune system is responsible for both conditions when they exist simultaneously.

Those who have taken large amounts of antibiotics, birth control pills, or corticosteroids, and those who have immune deficiencies, are thought to be more susceptible to yeast overgrowth. Treatment consists of medication and dietary modification. Medications include Nystatin, Nizoral (ketaconazole) and Diflucan (fluconazole); these medications are sometimes used in combination. (Liver studies should be done when PWCs are taking Nizoral or Diflucan.) Over-the-counter anti-yeast/antifungals are available but their efficacy is uncertain. Although some doctors treat many or all of their CFIDS patients with these remedies, others have not found them to be helpful.

PREDICTIONS

Although a cure is not known and may never be discovered, treatment of CFIDS is available and new medications are undergoing therapeutic trials in informal and formal scientific studies. All PWCs are guinea pigs in the sense that each treatment tried successfully or unsuccessfully adds to the fund of knowledge for treating CFIDS.

Treatment efforts in the future will be enhanced by our growing understanding of the immune system and ways in which we can influence immune system and neurological functioning. New drugs known as biological response modifiers, and lymphokine therapy in particular, treat immune system and neurological abnormalities and offer exciting future treatment possibilities for CFIDS and other immune disorders.

Chapter 12

◆

Coping with CFIDS

No matter how fragile the human body, the human
spirit can take just about anything.
            Cheri Register, *Living with Chronic Illness*

IN *THE HEALING HEART*, Norman Cousins discussed the
distinction between treatment and healing processes. The treatment process consists of various interventions of which the
body is not capable, the use of "outside" resources. Healing is
the patient's realm—using the body's own capabilities, since
healing is a natural drive of the body.

"I know there's no magic bullet," I wrote in my journal,

> I really want this problem to be solved by finding and eradicat-
> ing the "culprit." But I know there's more in me that needs to
> be taken care of. In general, I need to learn self-care, in all
> ways. My goal is integration of the physical, emotional, and
> spiritual. What I believe, my lifestyle, diet, friends . . . and the
> big questions. How do I choose to live? How can I best take
> care of myself? How can I find balance in my life? I never
> knew illness would raise such fundamental, difficult issues.
> The hunt for the magic bullet was simpler. I want life to be
> easy and simple, but it's complex and difficult.

I resisted the concept of "myself" as the most important resource. This notion placed too much responsibility on me for something I felt was beyond my control. I wanted the answers to come from "out there," but at the same time I didn't want to be a passive victim waiting for a gallant rescue. In time I have come to view this proposition as a cooperative one. The role of researchers and pharmaceutical companies is to keep searching for causes, effective remedies and, ultimately, cures. Simultaneously, I can maximize my internal resources both for coping with this illness and helping my body to rest and heal.

The complex interaction of factors that contribute to the development of illness (genetics, environmental influences, emotional factors, and lifestyle) suggests that the healing process is equally complex. Obviously we cannot change our genetic makeup, and most of us are not in a position to engage in scientific research, but we do have choices to make regarding belief systems, lifestyle, and the ways in which we deal with our emotions. Those of us who play an active part in our quest for coping will be more successful.

In a questionnaire I asked PWCs to list the treatments and healing modalities that they found helpful and not helpful. In assessing such treatments as medications, herbs, vitamins, and other "externals," the response to each was divided; some found these treatments helpful and some did not. However, such interventions as rest, positive attitude, relaxation/imaging tapes, religious faith, and stress reduction techniques were listed as helpful by all who mentioned them.

In a lecture on October 28, 1987, in Mesa, Arizona, Bernie Siegel, M.D., described characteristics of long-term AIDS survivors:

> acceptance of the diagnosis, but not as a death sentence
> personal coping system
> altered lifestyle for coping
> cooperation with their physicians
> commitment to life
> sense of meaningfulness and purpose in life
> supportive contact with other patients

assertiveness

self-nurturance

open communication regarding their needs

open communication regarding their feelings about their
    illness

Cancer patients who recover are fighters rather than victims;
they display anger and other feelings and maintain vitality.
They retain a sense of purpose; they reject the illness and
maintain a support system.

We can learn from these "successful" patients with other
illnesses to mobilize our own resources, especially our belief
systems. We can remain self-reliant to whatever degree possible,
maintaining a sense of adequacy and self-esteem. Rather than
resign ourselves to illness, we can learn to accommodate it as
best we can while striving toward improved health.

HOPE AND POSITIVE EXPECTATION

Hope is a strength-enhancing quality that is important to our
overall coping effort. Hope can be developed but it cannot be
manufactured or purchased. Unrealistic hope creates disappointment and lessens our chances of developing realistic hope
—the belief that we can endure and improve, and that the way
we feel now need not be forever.

Paula says:

> Mentally, I think I can affect my health by working at it,
> thinking more positive things, using positive visualization.
> Who knows how it works, but I think we can . . . . People with
> the will to live can overcome things that other people just
> give up on. People come back from near death to become
> marathon bicyclists. The rest of us just lead lives of quiet
> desperation.

"I have learned never to underestimate the capacity of the
human mind and body to regenerate—even when the prospects
seem most wretched. The life-force may be the least understood

force on earth," wrote Norman Cousins in 1979, emphasizing the importance of expanding our self-imposed limits and striving toward regeneration. By 1989, Cousins' belief in the positive role of hope and positive expectations had expanded. In *Head First* he emphasized the need for a positive patient-doctor relationship, reassurance ("the human apothecary"), a sense of purpose, hope, faith, love, determination and playfulness—which he considered "powerful biochemical prescriptions."

Other physicians, including Drs. Hans Selye, Bernie Siegel, Andrew Weil, Norman Shealy, and Stuart Berger, have written about the role of the positive emotions in determining our psychophysiological responses to illness—the powers of hope and positive expectations versus remaining stuck in anger, prolonged depression, despair, blame, hatred, and bitterness. Clinging to burdensome grievances becomes self-destructive; the negative emotions, like other forms of stress, rapidly cause an exacerbation of CFIDS symptoms, as PWCs have learned from experience.

Why are all these doctors writing about hope rather than microbes and medication? In ways that seem mysterious, love, positive beliefs, and spirituality mobilize the immune system and reinforce the notion that healing is indeed a remarkably complex process.

Psychoneuroimmunology (PNI), a relatively new branch of science with ancient roots, is likely to be the medical wonder-child of the twenty-first century. All body systems are inextricably connected; every part of the brain, psyche, immune system, respiratory system and other systems is in constant interaction; a change in any one part will affect the entire organism. Chemical messengers dash around madly inside us influenced no less by emotions than by medications and other so-called physiological events. Imagine a delicately balanced mobile: a tap on any part will affect all other parts as the mobile is set in motion, seeking to restore equilibrium. Once balance has been restored, the mobile once again comes to rest. Each part has played a role in restoring balance.

Still, many (probably most) doctors remain skeptical because they have been trained to believe that intervention at the physiological level (which is primarily what they do) holds the answers. Acknowledging the need to reduce stress and to eat and exercise sensibly, they are nonetheless guilty of underrating the innate healing potential of the human body, the role of the mind and emotions in so-called physical processes. Body parts are tangible; thoughts and beliefs are not. The ways in which the two interact are not yet well understood, making it easy to underestimate of the power and significance of mind-body interaction.

In our personal exploration it is important to examine our belief systems to determine if they are working for or against us. Hopelessness is a harmful medicine; hope, although not a cure-all, enables our bodies to mobilize toward healing.

In *The Mile-High Staircase*, Toni Jeffreys described alternating hope and despair, her unwillingness to be a passive victim, her need to fight, and her determination to remain optimistic despite discouraging setbacks. "We can be logical only up to the point where optimism and hope take over," she wrote. "That is both the limitation and the saving grace of the human condition."

Illness is a horrible catastrophe and a challenge in which hope and despair battle like archenemies. It's a juggling act. Hope takes over only to be replaced periodically by desperation and panic as exacerbations occur. How can we maintain faith that all will be well when symptoms rage and emotions run wild? Hope flees in the face of isolation, depression, anxiety, and an inability to feel "normal," as defined by past characteristics and behavior. The loss of control and our inability to trust our body to respond predictably or productively cause doubt—in ourselves, in others, and in the concept that things can ever be made right again. How can we dare to be hopeful when everything seems to be going wrong?

I wrote in my journal:

People say, "Things could be worse." We know they're right, but what good does it do? It's hard for me to be joyous because I don't have leprosy or cancer, but I still resent what I *do* have. Is it a crime to feel sorry for myself? I feel sorry for others who have CFIDS—why not me? People talk about "pity parties," an expression that makes me shudder. The concept heaps guilt on top of self-pity on top of pain. Why shouldn't I feel sorry for myself? This is a shitty illness. Why shouldn't I complain? It's a cheap hobby. People say, "Keep your chin up." I can't always do that. I feel better when I am able to be optimistic, and I'm that way about 80% of the time, maybe . . . but when I'm at my worst, hope goes to hell, along with everything else that feels good. But I know I will feel better again, that the world will appear different . . . and I look forward to that time. I know it's not possible to feel hopeful all the time, but it helps to know hopefulness will return.

So how do we "get" hope? How can we develop and maximize it? Anything that might work is worth trying. For some, part of the answer is spiritual belief, which does not necessarily mean organized religion, but rather our way of regarding life, the world, our purpose, and our ability to find peace and happiness. We examine our beliefs about life through reading, discussion, meditation, and self-exploration. We may not find ultimate conclusions or discover any earth-shattering cosmic truths but we can discover inner sources of positive belief.

Although a Pollyanna approach is not always possible or desirable, we can search for the measure of good in all people, events, and circumstances. I'm not talking about "faking it," putting on a happy face and pretending that everything is fine, but instead about embarking upon an exploratory process that can reveal various facets of our experiences. The black-and-white "all good or all bad" approach blocks the open, creative perceptions of which we are all capable.

The following suggestions have been used successfully by PWCs:

✦ Focus on "right now." The Alcoholics Anonymous approach, one day at a time, can be remarkably helpful. For example, rather than viewing myself as totally and irrevocably deprived and ripped off, it is helpful to realize that there are things I can't do *right now*. I believe that I will be able to do them at some unspecified time in the future.

Now isn't forever. Most things are temporary; life's only constant is its unpredictability.

✦ Plan something to look forward to, an event that is not likely to be jeopardized by a downward health swing. Have short-term goals that are simple and achievable in order to create a feeling of accomplishment. Break down large tasks into smaller components and take them one step at a time.

✦ When we focus on our deprivations, which is natural, we need to be aware of our blessings as well—not either/or but a balance of both. We forget how many things we have to be grateful for. Is the glass half empty or half full? We can learn to appreciate the small stuff—the beauty of sunlight captured in a prism, a child's smile, a funny movie.

✦ We have moment-by-moment decisions to make that affect our health. Deciding to rest when necessary rather than foolishly pushing on can help avoid a "crash." We don't choose feelings but we do choose behaviors.

✦ Continuing to explore healing and treatment alternatives leads us to those that seem most promising and least risky. If one fails, there are many others to consider.

✦ The advice "Learn to love yourself" sounds trite and self-ish. Despite its negative connotations, selfishness really means caring for ourselves and is a positive step in personal growth, unless carried to an extreme. Rather than criticize ourselves for our frailties (remember how we hated it when our parents did that?) let's focus on our strengths and individual worth. Our self-care will pay a bonus, allowing us to care more for others in turn. As the sum total of all of our individual ideas, feelings, values, likes, dislikes, characteristics, and traits, we are in some ways like all others and in some ways unique. We can and will endure this illness and deserve credit for making it as far as we have!

The biology of hope is no longer an abstract concept; learning to live well despite obstacles has a beneficial effect on immune functioning. The belief system has a direct influence on the healing system. Working toward peace of mind rather than perfect physical wellness ensures having an attainable goal. Hope cannot heal us but it can help the healing process. A determined attitude of confidence and letting go of blame will help us to move along the paths created by our positive expectations.

LIFESTYLE MODIFICATION

Activity level

Illness often tears a smoothly-functioning lifestyle to shreds. We go from one extreme to the other: from fully functioning to crashed, broken. When we begin to feel better, we start to try to do it all again, and then another crash. This cycle can continue indefinitely. I continued it long after I knew it was dysfunctional because of my denial that some lousy little virus (or whatever) had the power to devastate my chosen way of life. My tendency toward extremes compounded the problem and finally led me to seek a system that was more functional and less self-defeating: moderation—the "M" word. The concept of doing only what I was capable of in my compromised, limited state meant I could no longer pretend I could do anything and everything. It meant accomplishing less, resting more, and learning to balance priorities. I have hated this process, just as I dislike many of the things that are good for me; it's been a difficult yet valuable lesson in adaptation. I still don't like moderation too well, but I'm better at it, and it's helpful. I've decided not to stop living but to start living smarter and more flexibly.

Many of us are accustomed to being "on call" at all times: available to meet others' needs, to take care of things, to excel, to be busy constantly. We're not used to considering our own needs and priorities first. We've built our identities around taking care of others; we pride ourselves on being constantly achieving, giving. We don't recognize the imbalance inherent in this way of life until we get sick. Then we realize how much we've allowed others to depend on us and how we've come to expect unrealistic things of ourselves, allowing ourselves to be "enablers" by trying to be all things to all people. High expectations, self-pressure to do more and do it better, to push, to conquer and overcome obstacles, to work hard, never to disappoint ourselves or others, never to say "No"—this was normal! Anything less was unacceptable!

The opposite extreme, complete inactivity, can also be harmful. Having nothing to do and no reason to wake up in the morning is to have no meaning in one's life, no sense of purpose or value. It is devastating to one's self-esteem. Kyle reports that she feels better when she is able to work even part-time, "which didn't make any sense to me, except when I stayed home I just got weaker and weaker and more depressed, and my symptoms grew larger." Many PWCs are unable to work, but some can continue full-time or part-time. Work can offer a sense of purpose and validity. It may not be possible to continue a prior job or career, but finding meaningful activity is essential. We want to keep our bodies and minds functioning without pushing to a harmful degree.

We need to find flexible ways of continuing to function in accordance with our abilities, which can change weekly, daily, or hourly. It's difficult, but as long as we continue to abuse our bodies by pushing too hard, it's likely that any sort of treatment or healing efforts will fail. "Lifestyle adjustment [means] getting hold of the rheostat of your life and winding it down to 60% from what it was set before, which was sometimes at 120%," said Paul Cheney, M.D., at the CFS Convention in Oregon (November 1987). "As you wind it down to 60%, your functional capacity goes way up."

"I've learned to stop instead of pushing," says Paula:

> When I first came down with it, I kept pushing . . . . I've learned to back off. So the dishes don't get done. So the vacuuming doesn't get done this week. So the house isn't spotless. So what? So what? And I've never done that [before]. I've always been very hard-driving; I'm a perfectionist. Whatever I do, I had to be the best: the best mother, the best teacher, the best wife, the best whatever . . . the superwoman

syndrome. I had it all, but I lost it. Maybe if I moderate, I can gain back some of what I lost. I'm working part-time as a substitute teacher. I don't have to make an inspirational effort because I'm not the regular teacher; I have no preplanning and my days are short. While I'm working I usually feel better; I'm up; I'm doing something I enjoy doing. As long as I stick to my routine and I make sure I get the sleep I need and eat the proper foods and take care of myself, I do better. When I stop, it's real easy to get depressed.

Paula found that if she deviated substantially from her routine, she tended to overdo, under-rest, and crash:

My energy is like a basket. I have a basketful of energy; that's all the energy I have in the world. If I waste my energy on anger, then I don't have the energy to do something else. I try to control my temper, try to mellow out. I'm learning to use moderation in all facets of my life. I don't go to the extremes that I used to go to. It probably makes me an easier person to live with.

"My personal style won't change. I can't go from Type A to being totally mellow," says Bill. "I've had a lot of trouble with relaxation. I've been working and walking. I really need to sit down and reschedule my life." Bill created a system in which he could continue to work when he felt able, and he learned to delegate. He felt fortunate to have this degree of flexibility in his work—flexibility that he had never allowed himself in the past.

Betty described learning to rest:

I made out schedules for the course of a day. I make sure I rest, I mean bedrest. I know how to rest now. I watch TV sometimes and go to staff meetings every now and then, but not too often. [My boss] told me I could always be rehired, but I'm going to give myself a year. I need that break. I want to make sure that I don't get too overtired or sick. I want to keep a positive attitude. I want to lick this thing. I'm not pushing myself at all.

We need to regard energy reserves as a checking account. If we keep writing checks without making any deposits, we go into credit reserve. We tend to deplete the energy balance without giving thought to replenishing it and then are astonished when it's gone and we've crashed again. ("What do you mean I'm overdrawn? I still have checks left!") Balancing work and rest is difficult because our physical and emotional status keeps changing. Some days we can do a few things; other days, nothing at all. Sometimes we require frequent rest periods between activities and then feel rejuvenated. At other times we don't feel rejuvenated if we've rested for a week! Pushing harder won't help; it makes things worse. Adaptation is difficult but possible. Adapting doesn't mean giving in, being a wimp or a coward, but learning to be sensible, learning what to give up and what to continue—and to what degree. "It's like budgeting energy," said Yolanda. "I have so much for that day, and once it's gone, that's it. I know if I want to do a certain activity, I'd better not be cleaning the house ahead of time." She described having found new ways of doing things a little bit at a time.

CFIDS comes with a warning: adjust your life to this illness, or it will overcome you. That means sensible, flexible scheduling: saying "no" and "maybe" in response to requests, at least some of the time; reduced work load; increased rest and leisure. Rather than viewing CFIDS as an adversary against which to wage a futile war, learning to adapt (to choose activities wisely and to set limits) is more functional in the long run.

I used to carry a full patient load as a psychologist, teach college classes, and present frequent seminars and workshops. All that time I wished I had more time to complete further graduate studies and to write. After the onset of CFIDS I continued to work as I had before for as long as I could, becoming sicker and sicker. I didn't want to give up anything, but I finally realized I had painted myself into a corner and would need to either apply for disability benefits or cut way back on my activity level, neither of which was my style. Finally, I settled with myself: no teaching, two or three workshops a year, fewer lectures, and a decreased counseling load. It was difficult to give up so much of the work I love to do but I didn't have to give it all up. I am increasingly able to add to my load but ever cautious. In the meantime I use my "feeling good" times to write and my "down times" to rest. I still resent the down times, but I've learned to live with them. For me this has been a dramatic transformation. I've decided I'd never want to be as busy with "have-to's" as I was back then. I enjoy the flexibility and the time to write when I am able. I still hate this illness, but I've learned how to make some positive changes in my outlook and lifestyle.

Sleep and rest

Although some PWCs are confined to bed on a daily basis, most are able to be active to some extent. There is no formula for determining the optimum rest/activity ratio, which varies over time. Resting must be a priority. Some doctors speculate that insufficient rest will prolong the course of the illness as well as increase symptom severity.

Many of us have not learned how to rest, to turn off all outside stimuli and relax fully. We equate rest with sitting or lying down, but have not learned the relaxation skills to provide quality rest. Frequent rest periods throughout the day, or at least one rest between morning and afternoon activities, are usually beneficial, as is the use of relaxation tapes.

Although some people report that they are unable to get through the day without at least one nap, others find themselves unable to sleep at night if they have napped during the day. We must each establish our own sleep rhythms and learn what our patterns are, noting that they change over time. Sleep disturbances are common among PWCs: sleeping too much, being unable to fall asleep, having strange and vivid dreams or nightmares, frequent awakenings, or sleeping many hours without feeling refreshed. Getting to sleep may be facilitated by light reading or watching television at bedtime, hot baths shortly before bedtime, the use of relaxation tapes (see Chapter 14), and medications as discussed in Chapter 11.

Stress reduction

People boast of their achievements and conquests, but not about setting limits on their activity levels. Our society awards medals for accomplishing the most, the best, the fastest. We scorn those who take it easy—while we secretly envy them. A high-stress lifestyle is trendy; we are supposed to do it all, handle the pressure, juggle the roles. Our bodies aren't built to withstand such constant wear and tear. Just as cars that are driven constantly without stopping for maintenance or refueling will conk out, so will our bodies. It's time for a different, more sensible approach. Most of us weren't going to win a Nobel Prize anyway.

We need to be selective in our activities and issues, separating events within our control from those beyond it. We need to decide on a case-by-case basis whether to take an active or passive approach, determining what to fight against and what to accept. And when we can't change events, we still have the power to alter our responses to them. Stress cannot be avoided, but its effects can be minimized. It's a matter of degree. For a CFIDS patient to work full-time, to be an involved parent, and then expect to have energy left over for volunteer work and a busy social life is clearly unrealistic. It's probably unwise for even a healthy person to set up such a demanding schedule. Priorities must be set. In order to lower stress levels we need to examine and modify our unrealistic notions of what "normal" is for us *now*.

The following are suggestions for minimizing stress levels:

Establish realistic priorities and goals. You don't have to do it all; you don't have to do anything. Allow the way you are feeling to decide how much you can handle. Dump the "shoulds." No one's keeping score, and martyrs aren't awarded medals.

Manage time effectively. Develop a sense of your endurance level and times when you function best, and build your schedule accordingly. Don't take on more than you can reasonably handle. If anything, take on too little; you can always add more to a minimal schedule if you are able. It's easier than building a too-full schedule from which you must eliminate things.

Delegate tasks others can do.

Say "no" to inappropriate requests or to anything that's not in your best interests. Recognize that saying "no" is not the rejection of another person but simply the refusal of a request. Too often we equate being a people pleaser with being a "good person." You can be a good person by taking care of yourself—by setting limits and doing for others only what you are reasonably able to do.

Make requests. Ask others to do specific things that would be helpful to you. Remember, they, too, have the right to say "no," so allow them to assume responsibility for their responses to your requests. You know it feels good to help others; grant them the same privilege by allowing them to help you. Ask directly; don't hint or complain (e.g., "I'd appreciate your picking the kids up this afternoon," rather than "I'm so tired; I don't know how I'll ever be able to pick up the kids"). When we drop hints and others don't get the messages or act on them, we become needlessly hurt and resentful. Avoid this type of manipulative behavior by making direct requests.

Avoid total inactivity. Don't give up everything; total inactivity is stressful, too. Find a balance, a reasonable load. This may take some exploration, and the balance may change from time to time. Try to remain flexible, using energy as available.

Reprogram your thinking. If you're "doing a number" on yourself, being internally critical and blaming of yourself for your imperfections, examine the self-messages with which you beat yourself up. You shouldn't say anything to yourself that you wouldn't say to a close friend. Such statements as "I should be perfect," "Others should always approve of me," and "I should take care of others' problems for them" are just a few examples of negative, irrational self-messages which flourish with low self-esteem.

The following are examples of irrational CFIDS-related self-messages:

I'm too lazy

I should accomplish more

I shouldn't rely upon others

I'm just a weakling, I can't handle anything any more

I shouldn't feel the way I do

I should have gotten over this by now

I'm not supposed to have special needs

I'm just giving in to this; I'm not fighting hard enough

Such messages are irrational and damaging. They can, however, be reformulated. Many contain a grain of truth that has become terribly distorted. "I'm too lazy" can be modified into the more rational message "I feel fatigued." "I should accomplish more" can be restated as "I wish I could accomplish more, but that isn't realistic right now." "I can't handle anything" can become "It's very hard for me to cope with events when I'm feeling ill." List your irrational messages and then formulate rational alternatives. The input of others can help you to accomplish this.

"Before, the house had to smell like Pine-Sol; everything had to be clean. I used to have beautiful rose bushes. Everything looked perfect," says Betty. She talked over her "laziness" with her husband, her guilt that she no longer provided a showcase home for her family. "My husband said, 'So what?' My kids didn't care. It didn't bother me like it had before." Betty received her family's permission, and finally her own, to take better care of herself than she did of the house. Realize that the worst that can happen if a particular job goes undone is usually not too terrible after all.

Another bonus: our feelings are based not on external events but on our interpretation of those events, which are our self-messages. Reformulating irrational self-messages into rational ones causes the negative feelings to change and self-esteem to soar.

"I've worked real hard on not judging myself," says Paula. "I read about 'shoulds' and 'musts' and my whole life passed before me. So I worked hard on those shoulds and am learning not to put myself down. Any time you come across a should, it's usually from the outside. 'You should do this for your mother.'" Realizing how many of her self-expectations and messages stemmed from the manipulative and demanding behavior of others helped Paula to talk less judgmentally to herself and learn to set realistic limits. "When my mother says, 'If you were a good daughter, you would . . . ,' I say, 'Then I'm not a good daughter,' which brings her up short. Then she'll realize what she's done. It took me a long time to learn to do it." Talking rationally to ourselves gives us permission to appreciate our value and to behave more appropriately by freeing us from distorted, hurtful messages.

Problem solve. Identify personal problems and seek solutions. Reading self-help books, keeping a journal, and talking with others can be helpful. If you tend to blow things out of proportion, to turn minor events into catastrophes and then live in fear of dire consequences, seek the two things that will help you to feel better: information and reassurance. For example, if your fears are illness-related, read information about CFIDS, and ask others for the reassurance you need. Also become aware of the irrationality of some of your fears; again, examining self-messages can help.

Give up the "rescuer role". If you habitually attempt to rescue or control others (a trait called codependency), recognize the futility of this behavior. Too often we work at "fixing" others, spending lots of energy attempting to understand them, getting them to understand themselves, and causing them to change. The result is that others do not change and we have wasted valuable energy. The only person you can effectively take care of is yourself. Direct your efforts toward self-care. You will continue to care *about* others, but to stop trying to take care *of* them (which is taking over their job). Allow others to assume responsibility for self-care, just as you are doing. In taking this approach you may feel as if you're abandoning others, but you're really doing them and yourself a favor. Give others credit for having the ability and the responsibility to take care of themselves. A good rule of thumb (but one difficult to follow) is never to do for others what they could and should do for themselves. Attempting to control the lives of others means taking on a stressful burden that is not beneficial for either party. It's definitely not good for your health.

Find Support. Share with others—those who have CFIDS and those who don't. PWCs can provide valuable understanding and support; they can relate directly to your situation. Those without CFIDS cannot understand in the same way but can add a valuable outside perspective and keep you from getting totally caught up in the illness. To internalize your feelings seems heroic, but it's foolish. Reach out.

Pamper Yourself. Do things that make you feel good. Don't deny yourself what you want and need because you're ill. It's not your fault you're ill and you certainly don't deserve to be punished. Take a bubble bath or cuddle up with your pet. Watch television. Read a good book if your brain is working or a trashy one if it isn't. One former ice skater spends her time watching videotapes of ice skaters to keep in touch with her favorite activity. Another PWC loves to cook. She spends most of the day in bed and gets up in time to cook dinner for her family, an enjoyable activity for her. Another gave up bike riding because it was too strenuous but discovered her long-neglected guitar in the garage and began to play it again.

Avoid what's bad for you. Avoid situations that tend to be stressful to avoid relapses. Drastic changes of any kind should be avoided or minimized. Air travel is problematic for many patients, whether because of toxic fumes, recirculated air, altitude, or abrupt climate changes. Some avoid air travel entirely, and some continue, allowing a few days after a trip to rest. Discover your exacerbation "triggers" and avoid them.

Laugh! Although there is no hard evidence, humor is a restorative, healing force with beneficial physiological effects. Laughter can help one to let go of negative emotions and reduce anxiety levels. It is believed to have beneficial effects on the immune system as well. Norman Cousins used laughter to help diminish pain, induce sleep, and promote healing during a serious illness, and extolled the benefits of laughter in his books

Anatomy of an Illness and *Head First*. "Illness is not a laughing matter," he wrote. "Maybe it ought to be" (1989, p. 313).

My ability to laugh is a health barometer and an important coping mechanism. My sense of humor hibernates when I'm feeling ill; I worry about myself when I take life too seriously. When I'm very ill my sense of humor seems irretrievably lost, but it returns eventually. Sometimes the right person or situation brings it out of hiding. Then I feel like me again.

Seek out the people you enjoy. Put yourself in the company of people who are funny and uplifting, either in person or by telephone. Avoid the "downers" and the "needies"—especially at times when you are down and needy.

Holidays: Go easy. Don't build up unrealistic expectations (Waltons' Syndrome). Perfect families exist only on TV, not in real life. Don't knock yourself out—let others pitch in; tell them what you need. If you have a rule that you must cook everything from scratch, forget it—use a mix or don't cook at all. Delegate. A postholiday crash is a horror to be avoided at all costs. It's just not worth it. Others should be understanding, but if they're not, it isn't your problem. Self-care must be a priority. You won't be much fun if you work yourself into a grouchy relapse. Enjoy the holidays as much as you can; sing "I'm dreaming of a dead virus" and "All I want for Christmas is some en-er-gy." If you lack energy to sing, then hum.

Learn to relax. Many people don't know how. There are many ways to practice relaxation; experiment with techniques to determine what is most effective for you. Relaxation is a skill to be learned and practiced like any other. Its beneficial effects are felt both immediately and over time, at the emotional, spiritual, and physiological levels. Individual responses vary, and there is no one correct method or technique that is superior to others. Read about various techniques and try them on your own, purchase a prerecorded audiocassette (see Appendix A), or consult a stress management clinic, a psychotherapist, or a physician specializing in stress management.

In most relaxation exercises the individual assumes a comfortable position in an environment free of distractions. Muscle relaxation and deep breathing are employed; affirmations or certain phrases are repeated internally; and images of healing, relaxing settings, and/or immune enhancement are developed. The individual returns slowly to the environment. Relaxation exercises are generally practiced once or twice a day for about twenty minutes.

The use of guided imagery is based on the theory that an individual's ability to imagine and feel a positive outcome can help to create it. Carl Simonton, M.D., Stephanie Matthews Simonton, and Bernie Siegel, M.D., have used guided imagery extensively with cancer patients and have found it to be very helpful.

Imagery clearly has application in the treatment of CFIDS. It provides a time-out period during which one can clear the mind and look inward to develop insights, create peaceful feelings, and encourage self-healing, producing emotional changes that in turn create internal change in neurochemistry and physiology.

My images vary. Sometimes I visualize my thymus gland receiving messages from my hypothalamus to produce lots of healthy T-cells, or even cartoon-like warriors in battle—_POW! BAM!_ The images can be scientific or goofy, whatever feels comfortable, so long as your images are compatible with your belief system. The more appropriate and well-defined the image, the more effective the imagery will be.

Biofeedback is a training process that takes place over a period of weeks or months. It employs equipment that monitors bodily functions, indicating one's level of relaxation, such as muscle tension and hand temperature, and offers feedback in the form of noises or flashing lights to signal progress toward the desired response. Relaxation techniques are used along with biofeedback instruments, which simply monitor functioning while the individual learns to relax. The patient develops a sense of control over bodily functions that are usually beyond conscious control. Biofeedback is also helpful for treating certain symptoms such as headache and body pain.

Meditation is the process of focusing one's attention on a bland stimulus in order to clear the mind and produce a sense of inward calm. Tuning out distractions and lowering body arousal brings a sense of quietness and peace, which feels good and is thought to bring about positive psychological/physiological changes. Several types of meditation are taught. Some use a mantra, or a meaningless phrase for focus; others use a one-syllable word such as "one," or words related to the desired outcome, such as "calm and relaxed." Deep breathing and turning the mind off are the commonalities among all types, which may be learned from a trainer, a psychotherapist, books, or audiotapes. Goals include relaxation, stress reduction, spiritual development, expansion of the mind, and heightened creativity.

Autogenic Training is a form of relaxation that relies on passive concentration accompanied by certain phrases related to a series of specific exercises. These are aimed toward the creation of bodily sensations, such as feelings of warmth and heaviness and slowed breathing. Mastering these highly structured exercises requires continual practice. As with meditation, individual instruction, group instruction, or materials used on one's own can teach this skill.

Hypnosis is frightening to some people whose only exposure to it has been watching people on television acting like ridiculous barnyard animals. Such simplistic, erroneous notions about the powers of hypnosis are misleading. Hypnosis is the achievement of an altered state of consciousness in which the unconscious mind plays a central role. Hypnosis taps the neural links between mind and body—the psyche and the soma. In this context we attempt to convert words, ideas, sensations, beliefs, and expectations into the physiological healing process.

A hypnotized individual is in full control at all times and will refuse to do anything objectionable or harmful. It is important to work with a reputable hypnotherapist with training credentials, experience, and an approach with which the client is comfortable. Self-hypnosis can be learned by working with a hypnotherapist, using commercially marketed cassette tapes, or practicing exercises from reputable self-help books.

Massage may provide benefits such as increased relaxation, decreased pain, improved circulation, and other positive physiological and emotional effects. Massages may be given by professionals (use a reliable referral source), or someone you know may be willing to learn massage techniques.

Exercise promotes cardiovascular fitness, strengthens muscles, burns calories, and fights depression. Some PWCs report that mild exercise produces increased energy and mental alertness, which may be caused by the production of energizing hormones called catecholamines. Exercise has been speculated to enhance immune functioning. It provides a temporary escape from problems and creates a sense of accomplishment, a self-esteem boost. One PWC reports that he walks "just to be out in public. It makes me feel like I'm part of life again."

However, exercise is not appropriate for all PWCs. Medical advice, common sense, and a trial-and-error process help determine its advisability. If you have not exercised in some time, start slowly, perhaps with only a brief warm-up routine or stretching exercises. Yoga, t'ai chi, or low-impact aerobics may be tolerable and helpful. Stop exercising when you _begin_ to feel fatigued; don't wait for exhaustion to set in. If exercise makes you feel worse, discontinue it.

I used to jog, hike, and play racquetball. My body tells me not to do those things any more, and I've learned to listen. I've goofed; once during a remission I felt good enough to play racquetball for an hour. Then I crashed, hard, for several weeks. It wasn't worth it. Now I do stretching exercises when I feel up to it.

Creating a New Life Philosophy

Illness offers us new opportunities whether we want them or not, and forces us to examine issues that would otherwise be left unexplored. No longer able to view the world in accustomed ways, we question the meaning of life—specifically, views of our own lives.

If we perceived ourselves as passive victims before becoming ill, this view may be significantly increased with the onset and continuation of CFIDS. Learning to view ourselves as active, influential (but not omnipotent!) forces in the course of our lives creates the opportunity to identify options and make positive choices.

What really matters? Our experience with CFIDS teaches us that many of the things that mattered before aren't really that important. Thinking ahead, "Will this issue be important three or six months from now?" we realize most things don't matter that much.

Our value systems undergo change; we may become less materialistic and more in touch with health issues, the importance of relationships with family and friends, and spiritual beliefs. We come to place greater value on self-care. We become more human, loving, aware of people and things around us, and fully alive, as weird as that sounds when we feel half-dead.

Spirituality in the sense of organized religion or development of one's own belief system through reading, talking with others, and meditating is helpful to many PWCs. Some have stated that their religious/spiritual beliefs allowed them to get through the CFIDS ordeal, which involves a great deal of questioning and attempting to understand life/death, illness/wellness, and other issues in a clearer way. As prior beliefs are questioned, involvement with a traditional or nontraditional belief system is a source of great comfort.

We learn to rely less upon the opinions and beliefs of others as a result of their misunderstanding of CFIDS and our ensuing lifestyle changes. Thus we come to rely more fully upon ourselves and to respect the resources that have enabled us to learn, cope, and survive. We learn that our own approval has the most value.

No longer able to rely upon former goals and life expectations, we learn to value and live in the moment, to take advantage of "right now." It's too late for yesterday, although we remain nostalgic for the way things used to be, and too soon for tomorrow, which is made especially unpredictable by radical fluctuations in health. Today is all we've got to work with. "I used to be into 'tomorrow,'" says Betty. "I mean long-term everything. I was so computerized and programmed." Now Betty is doing much less but appreciating each moment more fully.

Illness offers an opportunity to develop a new sense of purpose. A retired college professor who had always wanted to learn charcoal drawing enjoys his new-found talent. Some PWCs have adopted CFIDS as their primary cause, writing for newsletters, facilitating support groups, or becoming politically involved.

Chronic illness teaches us (once again) that life is not fair. And we try to come to terms with that truth, while resenting it fully. We are angry that life is unfair. Bad things do happen to good people. No matter how strong or competent we may be, we can't make this illness go away. We are forced to live with it and deal with it. More hard lessons.

As our ability to function waxes and wanes, our lives gain and lose meaning. Everything is up for grabs; life becomes chaotic. But from the chaos can emerge transformative insights and understandings. As we meet the major challenge of leading meaningful lives despite severe limitations, our perceptions are permanently altered. We learn to identify and rid ourselves of extraneous baggage and focus on what really matters. The process of learning to live and love more fully is necessary to our individual and collective survival.

FEELINGS

What are feelings anyway? You can't see them or find the right words for them; they defy logic. And yet they're undeniably there. Our feelings vary unpredictably, interspersed with denial or numbness borne of a need to push difficult emotions away.

We are taught that hiding emotions, or better still, not having them in the first place, is a sign of maturity and strength. ("Bi-ig girls, they don't cry-iy-iy," went the song.) If we can't deny feelings, we attempt to justify them with elaborate explanations or apologize for them. I'll bet that 80% of my patients cry in counseling sessions at one time or another and most of them apologize. People are *supposed* to express feelings in a psychologist's office and yet many of them need permission because of our cultural taboo.

I'm not advocating that we announce our current emotional status every thirty minutes. It's natural to have feelings and it's normal to express them. Rules to the contrary don't make any sense. We have no choices about what feelings to have; as human beings, we're going to have all of them and often unpredictably. Our rational minds will say, "No need to feel upset about *that*," while our emotions have other plans. We do have a choice, though, about how to deal with those emotions behaviorally—how we express them.

Emotions don't have to be justified. They are not to be judged. Sometimes we choose to conceal them, at least temporarily, but any strong feeling will ultimately need to be expressed in some way. However uncomfortable, feelings are a manifestation of being human. We might as well accept them and learn to handle them the best we can.

PWCs experience fear regarding the illness and its possible implications and complications. The procedures we have undergone, the new treatments we have tried, and the strange symptoms we have experienced are all frightening. There is so much that remains unknown, and the unknown is always scary. Expressing the fear and seeking both information and reassurance is enormously helpful. Consider talking with family, friends, and health care professionals about your fears. We may use humor to mask fear, which is healthy to a degree. It's a relief to be able to laugh at ourselves.

Anger is considered the most unacceptable emotion; we tend to equate it with shouting, belligerence, loss of control, and hurtful exchanges. It need be none of these. Anger is a natural emotion and can be expressed constructively, although many of us have never had role models for the healthy expression of anger. We're used to seeing anger displaced and have probably done so ourselves, blowing up at a child or spouse when we're really angry because we're sick. We often make the mistake of allowing angry feelings to control us because we don't realize the options we have for dealing with them. Anger means there's a problem that needs to be addressed and solved.

It begins with hurt or some other unexpressed feeling. When we are emotionally sensitive, as we are during CFIDS exacerbations, anger is close to the surface and can be easily triggered by minor events.

Why are we angry? We're angry that we're sick. That we're deprived. That we don't have energy. That we can't do what others can do, or what we used to do. We're angry that we've been singled out to be sick while other people are well. We're angry because we feel misunderstood by health care professionals, the media, and those close to us. We're angry because there's no cure. We're angry because we can't will CFIDS away, no matter how good we are. We're angry because we've lost so much. We're angry because we don't know if we can get back what we've lost. We're angry when others don't really listen to us or hear what we're trying to say. We're angry because we often can't express ourselves as we'd like to. We're angry because we're scared, lonely, and miserable. We're angry because our income is limited and our medical bills are huge. We're angry at ourselves because we don't know what to do to make ourselves well again. We're angry because our responsibilities and expectations continue although our energy does not. We're angry because we often don't like ourselves or accept our situation very well.

We have good cause to be angry, and need to find safe outlets for our anger. Some suggestions: express it, verbally or in writing, but not in an accusatory manner. Identify the problems and feelings that may have triggered the anger; when these are dealt with, the anger may dissipate. If you feel you may explode at someone (an act that you could later regret), get away temporarily and return when you are capable of a more reasonable discussion. Physical activity can be helpful, if possible. Try throwing darts, pounding a pillow, throwing unbreakable things, or yelling out loud when you are alone. Allow your anger to help you identify problem issues and work through them. Don't allow it to jeopardize your relationships with others; don't attempt to "punish" them or yourself. If you try to repress anger, it will turn to bitter resentment or to depression, two undesirable outcomes. So express it carefully, in a way that isn't belittling or damaging to others. Simply let them know how you feel. Warn your spouse or significant other when you are feeling anger in order to help them interpret your comments and actions.

Having watched a talk show about AIDS, Paula said:

[The AIDS patients] were talking about forgiving yourself; forgiving the people around you all the hurts and the angers, to allow you to love yourself. And if you let go of the anger and the fear, your body will start to heal itself. I sat there stunned . . . . It's going to take a lot of work to let go. I hadn't thought that much about loving myself . . . . I resent my body for having failed me. To forgive that and love myself [is] something foreign . . . . Releasing suppressed anger would give me energy.

Later, Paula noted that her difficulty in asking others to do things for her caused her to become "very demanding, very resentful, very angry, which caused [them] a lot of anger in response to me. What I was giving out was what was coming back."

Depression usually waxes and wanes; for some it remains constant. Depression is a result of being ill, suffering limitations and losses, and of distorted thinking which results in irrational self-messages. It's quite painful but natural to be depressed. Sometimes the depression occurs in reaction to an event, at other times it seems to sweep over one unexpectedly and is more difficult to accept because it's impossible to understand. What to do? Some hot tips: allow yourself to feel, to experience the depression. Allow it to run its course. Denying it and faking happiness can prolong the depression. Cry and feel sorry for yourself for a while; you will emerge from depression once you have gone through it. As difficult as it is to believe during a depressive episode, it's not forever. You really will feel good again. Identify other issues (problems, repressed emotions) that have triggered the depression and deal with them when you are able. It's okay and even helpful to cry. Tears are cathartic. One PWC described times when she was profoundly depressed but unable to cry. When the tears finally came, the depression lifted. We discussed "crying triggers," for example, certain songs or sad movies that would invoke tears to complete the cycle for her.

Plan things to look forward to whenever possible. Enlist the support of others, or if you need to be alone, try to communicate this so others won't feel rejected. (When you withdraw, people often think you're angry at them.) Learn what you can from the depression; for some reason, the most meaningful learning experiences are painful. Physical touch may help, as can some type of meaningful activity if you are up to it.

When I'm severely depressed I need to be left alone to feel lousy and get through it. When I'm just somewhat depressed I often undertake a chore I hate, which discharges some of the negative feelings and gives me a feeling of accomplishment. Or I force myself to call a friend, typically someone with an inane sense of humor—"Emergency! Restore my sanity, please!" Or I write a letter. No matter what the salutation says, I'm really writing to myself. I never mail these letters. I just say whatever is locked up inside. Some of these techniques may work for you.

Talking about feelings can help, even about feelings that have been talked about before. You can talk to yourself or talk with others. Let others know that your intent is only to express feelings and sort them out, that you're not expecting to be rescued or fixed. Let them know whether or not you want feedback; sometimes we just need to talk, and other times we want to hear reactions in order to develop new perspectives.

Keeping a journal serves several functions. One is catharsis: writing thoughts and feelings allows us to experience and clarify them in a new way and to find new meaning in them. As we write, we learn about ourselves. We should write only for ourselves but may later choose to share with others parts of what we have written. Blocked emotions will often surface; old baggage ("unfinished business") can be explored and laid to rest. A journal of events, reactions, thoughts, and feelings allows not only self-expression but also an opportunity to review the past by rereading. You will probably surprise yourself with newly developed insights and progress. A shy psychotherapy patient said very little during her early sessions although she was experiencing deep conflicts and insecurities. She began to keep a journal. Each week she'd shyly present her recent entries for me to read. Having communicated in writing about events, thoughts, and feelings she could not verbalize, she became able to talk about them.

Unexpressed feelings fester within, later popping out unexpectedly and often inappropriately. Repressed emotions may be damaging psychologically and physiologically to individuals and relationships. The constructive expression of feelings can enhance relationships, but the feelings themselves (not the other person, or the other person's feelings) must be the focus. Constructive emotional expression does not involve placing blame, labeling, or criticizing others.

GRIEVING: HANDLING LOSS

The process of grieving is a difficult and painful but necessary reaction to any significant loss. Healing cannot take place until the loss is mourned. We tend to think of losses as being death- or money-related, but there are many other types. CFIDS-related losses are: energy, vitality and enthusiasm, good health, ability to perform responsibilities and activities, certain roles, pleasure, motivation, predictability and control, income, self-esteem, some relationships, others' former attitudes toward us, jobs and/or careers, educational or training plans, leisure activities, plans, and dreams. We have literally lost vital parts of our lives and of ourselves. As Paula comments:

> All our plans for the future, all our dreams about what we were going to accomplish, that took a lot of effort, hard work and time, cannot come to pass because I can't do it now. All those great plans of accomplishing great things and making lots of money, the trips and vacations, and doing for the kids, having the material things we'd planned on, are all gone. Realizing that I'm going to have to put those aside and start from scratch again and build from where we are and from what I can do [is difficult].

There are several stages in the grieving process: denial, bargaining, anger, depression, and acceptance. We may experience the stages in order, skip around, omit certain stages entirely or return to one stage repeatedly. There's no right way to grieve, nor an easy one.

The **denial** stage is often experienced as a general numbness, reflecting our inability to absorb and deal with a painful experience all at once. We feel the difficulties and pain can't possibly happen to us. This illness just can't be real. To protect ourselves from being overwhelmed by the sudden impact, we numb out, allowing the hurt to surface and be absorbed gradually. During this stage we may tend to overdo in terms of activity level and then crash, often repeatedly, as we alternately deny and are reminded of our illness. Using humor or intellectualizing the problem may serve as buffers in this stage and can be helpful if used to help us survive this stage rather than keeping us stuck there.

During the **bargaining** phase we try to make deals with ourselves, our doctors, or with God. It's a promise to "be good" in exchange for restoration of what we have lost. "If I eat vegetables, deny myself junk food, if I listen to 'doctor's orders,' maybe I'll get back my good health in return." And there are the retrospective "if only's" . . . if only I had taken better care of myself, not gone on that long trip, not tried to do so much, not taken those antibiotics, not eaten junk food. We can get stuck in this stage or return to it periodically, but generally the bargaining stage is brief, if we experience it at all.

Anger! Much of the anger lies in the unfairness of a situation that's beyond our control. There's no responsible party, no single causative event, and no direct revenge to be taken. CFIDS shouldn't happen to us or to anyone. There should be a cure. Our suffering should be better understood by others. There should be more research. That all these things are true doesn't change anything. We are angry because we've been hurt and deprived. The anger stage is guilt-producing: not only are we more dependent on others, but sometimes we're not even *nice* to them. Others will tolerate and excuse some of our anger, but we need to channel it in nondestructive ways. Getting to and through the anger stage is a significant step toward recovery from emotional wounds.

Sadness/depression is the period of hurt that accompanies the full realization that what has happened is real and devastating. Hopelessness, helplessness, disappointment, isolation, and self-pity dominate the emotional scene. During this stage we may feel that our lives are over, we'll never feel good again, we are totally useless, everything has been taken away, no one understands, and there's nothing left to live for. As depression lifts, anger may resurface as the feelings are directed outward instead of inward.

Adaptation. "Ultimately chronic fatigue syndrome becomes a background fact of life, not a foreground obsession," wrote Karyn Feiden. Our losses become integrated into our lives. We give up trying to manipulate reality and accept the situation. We make peace instead of war. We adapt to a difficult situation and focus on what we can do, remaining painfully aware of what we cannot do. New strengths emerge. We stop living in the "if onlys," with what should be (if only I were well again, if only I had never gotten sick), and learn to live with what is. We begin to restructure our lives. CFIDS, we realize, is not the sole factor that defines us. We can live within its limitations and go on. We are able to focus outward again, to become aware of others and their needs. We are less afraid, more able to accept ourselves and others. We have learned to be flexible, for our very survival depends upon our ability to bend, to go with the flow. Rather than remain passive and stuck, we move forward, taking responsibility for the management of our lives. But our fears and doubts continue; acceptance is a matter of degree.

This process is lengthy and bumpy; there are no shortcuts. We bounce back and forth between stages, sometimes feeling we've arrived at the adaptation stage, only to find ourselves back in anger, denial, or depression. Having been there before makes it a little easier the second, third, or fourth time around. Knowing we've survived these stages before allows us to feel less trapped and overwhelmed by them.

COUNSELING

Remember the old movies in which the psychiatrist (a bearded man on the other side of the desk or couch) remained detached, aloof, stroking his beard and saying "uh huh" occasionally? And only crazy people went to see him, right? Since then there have been movies like *Ordinary People*, in which therapists are depicted as human beings who are trained to help people sort out issues and problem-solve. There used to be a great stigma attached to therapy, but seeking help has become more acceptable—even trendy in some circles. It's not a sign of weakness to seek professional help for coping with the devastating effects of CFIDS: life adjustment issues, depression, and anxiety. Therapy is a safe place to express feelings. It can feel good to have time for yourself, focusing solely on your needs without guilt about not meeting the needs of others. As Stephanie Simonton pointed out in *The Healing Family*, "It is not a sign of failure to seek a therapist but a willingness to grow."

Local and national support groups, physicians, and other PWCs can provide names of CFIDS-educated therapists. Many qualified therapists are only vaguely familiar with CFIDS and will need to become educated by PWCs. A therapist who is experienced in treating those with chronic illnesses will generally appreciate receiving CFIDS literature.

Other people may not understand or approve of your seeking psychological help. Their opinions are not your problem, but you may be negatively affected by their attitudes. If so, explain to them the basis for your decision but don't feel you must justify it.

A good fit between therapist and client is essential. If you feel understood and taken seriously and the therapist is supportive and growth-oriented, you have probably found someone with whom you will work well. If you have reservations, discuss them with the therapist to see if the problems can be solved. If not, you're the consumer; find another therapist with whom you feel more comfortable. If this process occurs repeatedly, examine your expectations; if they're unrealistic, you will never find someone who can meet them.

SUPPORT GROUPS

There are two main types of CFIDS support groups: larger, information-oriented groups at the state- or large city-level, and smaller emotional support groups. Larger organizations often operate CFIDS "hotlines" and distribute newsletters to members. Smaller therapy groups may be led by professionals or by PWCs, where the group's goal is to meet individual needs by sharing and interacting. Many PWCs participate in both types of groups.

In the group setting we are reminded that we do not suffer alone, that other PWCs share our struggle. Comfort, support, shared feelings, coping suggestions, exchange of information about treatment, and the opportunity to help others can be invaluable. As one CFIDS group participant said, "Joining this group is the best thing I ever did. Now I know I'm not crazy."

I conducted a CFIDS support group that met regularly for about eighteen months. Group size varied unpredictably because of health fluctuations. We discussed such topics as practical problem solving; life disruption and changes; dealing with the medical community; dropping the "I'm fine" facade; self-care; feelings regarding CFIDS, our lifestyles and limitations; coping and adaptation skills; communicating with family, friends, employers, and coworkers; seeking new meaning and opportunities; learning moderation; relaxation and healing techniques; identifying and changing irrational self-messages; and exchange of individual experiences and concerns.

Some patients report that although some group interaction is helpful, too much contact or negative contact causes further preoccupation with CFIDS. Bill says, "I have decided for the time being to divorce myself, where possible, from . . . support groups and reading the literature. I found that, after a while, these contacts were making me more obsessed with the illness." Such is often the case when complaining becomes the main focus of a group—a pitfall to be avoided. Talking to people who are sicker than we are or who have been sick for a longer time can fuel our pessimism. Conversely, talking with those who are doing really well can make us feel like failures, like losers in a competition. Supportive contact with other CFIDS patients needs to be balanced with people and things in the "well world."

COPING TECHNIQUES

The following summary list of suggestions has been compiled from patient reports, personal experience, books, and articles.

Learn moderation and self-pacing

Get adequate rest

Make self-expectations more realistic, reasonable and doable

Learn to "Go with the flow": do what you can, and let the rest go

Talk positively to yourself

Focus more on taking care of yourself and less on "fixing" others

Delegate responsibility

Ask for what you need (e.g., support, help, reassurance)

Seek to build and maintain healthy relationships with others

Let go of the need to accomplish constantly

Recognize and express emotions constructively: deal with depression and the grieving process; don't repress feelings

Recognize and seek to eliminate self-defeating behaviors

Develop a sensible nutrition/exercise program; exercise moderately if you can; don't force anything that doesn't feel good or right; don't push; take it very slowly

Learn to listen to your body; respect and understand its signals

Look for meaning and purpose in your life through doable activities and goals

Become aware of the things for which you are grateful

Learn to appreciate small pleasures

Learn to cope with an unpredictable future

Retain your sense of humor as much as possible

Examine your perspectives and life philosophy; determine what really matters to you

Learn to slow down and live in the moment—stop and smell the roses

Accept that life is not fair and that we must learn to do the best we can with what we have

Learn to be more patient, more flexible, less driven, less perfectionistic

Try to communicate frequently and productively with others

Communicate with yourself: keep a journal in which you can write all the things you're not willing or able to communicate with others

Identify and develop new resources

Give yourself credit for coping with a very difficult situation

Recognize that your primary job right now is getting well

Learn to put away the past (hurts, angers, resentments)

Use "now" as a standard, not how you used to be

Work on stress reduction

Seek positive relationships with physicians and other health care professionals

Respect your body's innate self-healing potential and attend to your body's needs

Learn about illness and wellness; ask questions, seek answers and new ideas

Educate those you love about your illness

Prioritize. As one PWC said, "If I can't do it, screw it!"

Don't define yourself solely in terms of the illness

Keep a calender of symptoms, activities, life changes, and medications, and try to find correlations or patterns to identify helpful and harmful factors

Take one step at a time

Do the things that make you feel good

Let go of as many "shoulds" as possible

Identify and deal with other life problems, which can compound the effects of illness

Don't compare your progress to that of others
Practice self-affirmations and healing imagery
Don't apologize for being ill or having limitations
Treat yourself with dignity and respect
Forgive yourself and others when you can. Throw guilt
   and blame out the window
Laugh!
Reach out to others: talk, hug, touch, love.

Chapter 13

◆

CFIDS
and Relationships

W HEN CFIDS DISRUPTS OUR LIVES, it affects those
with whom we are close as well. Relationships are altered by
changes in individuals. We experience the dual pull of wanting
to share our pain with others and wanting to pull away from
them into our cocoons. Others have the dual reaction of wanting to be understanding and helpful and wanting to escape from
the pain and helplessness of watching a loved one suffer.

We ask ourselves how much it's appropriate and safe to
confide in others and how to help them understand. We wonder how they can live with us and how much of our illness and
our ill behaviors they will tolerate before they leave us. We
wonder if caring will crumble in the face of adversity.

And as much as we try to share the experience with others,
we realize that this illness is ours alone. Others may be victims
of the fallout, but we bear the direct brunt. CFIDS changes us.
We need to understand our changes in order to cope productively
with changes in our relationships. We need the cooperation of
others in order to adapt and cope with our relationships.

Important people in our lives need to be educated regarding the illness and its effects so that they can better understand
what is happening. In deciding how much information to give

them, we should consider their roles in our lives and how much interest they have in CFIDS. Sources of information include medical literature, popular literature, books about CFIDS, discussions, and attendance at support group meetings. Some partners may want to read everything available, but most will generally be satisfied with a few articles. It's best to select those that present a lot of general information concisely, and which are at an appropriate reading level. Most people will probably not want to read detailed medical information but would like to know about the possible causes, effects and symptoms, the duration of the illness, and any theories regarding contagion (see Chapter 1).

We should also help others to understand that we also have greater needs than in the past. It is the responsibility of the PWC to identify these personal needs and ask others for appropriate help in meeting them. Others should act as supportive helpers rather than rescuers. The role of rescuer involves mindreading and inappropriate assistance, that is, doing for others what they should do for themselves. Rescuing may seem helpful and even heroic but it is neither. It is usually harmful to the PWC's self-esteem and puts both parties at risk of developing resentments. Giving advice is a form of rescuing and is generally not well received unless it is requested or clearly needed; otherwise it is likely to be viewed as an intrusion and disregarded. Caregivers need to sort out what is helpful from what is intrusive. In general, caregivers are most helpful when they offer help without pushing.

Clear communication is extremely important. Often, we want to be open but also feel we should say what the other person wants to hear, which can create barriers between people. We tend to "clean up" our statements to make them seem acceptable; in the process we censor our true feelings. Acknowledging these feelings can be scary and difficult, but relationships are enhanced when the freedom to express feelings openly is maximized. The notion that good people don't have "bad" feelings is a myth. We're not saints; we're real people with real feelings. Bottling up so-called unacceptable feelings causes them to fester—and to multiply.

Learning to communicate assertively is a good idea regardless of health status. Assertiveness means expressing one's ideas, feelings, and needs appropriately, not aggressively: asking for what we need, refusing inappropriate requests or demands, and making direct statements rather than hints. It allows people to communicate honestly without covering up or protecting one another. It enhances self-esteem and feelings of self-control, thus helping to combat depression.

Sexual relationships are affected by CFIDS. Many PWCs experience decreased sex drive, and males may experience impotence, the inability to have or maintain an erection. Certain medications as well as the illness itself may cause delayed orgasm, another source of frustration for PWCs. Lack of energy contributes to these sexual difficulties. Couples should communicate about the change in sexual frequency and other issues. Less frequent sex and less vigorous or satisfying sex is disappointing; individuals and couples feel deprived of intimacy. Adaptive measures, including cuddling without pressure for sex and less vigorous sexual activities, help to make up for the losses. If discussion and problem-solving attempts are unsuccessful, a sex therapist can help with CFIDS-related sexual issues.

GRIEF AND MOURNING

Couples and families, as well as individual PWCs, may feel a need to grieve. The losses they experience are many: financial hardship, familiar patterns and activities, ways of sharing responsibilities. In addition, those who care about the PWC will be affected personally by her or his losses as an individual. You may be able to grieve together, going through the process at the same pace, or you may arrive at different stages independently. Emotional sharing keeps loved ones in touch with each others' feelings and experiences. If emotional expression has been repressed or denied in the relationship in the past this sharing will be doubly difficult, but it is still necessary so that people don't grow apart.

Grieving and rebuilding allow new strengths and interests to emerge. Just as we need to grieve with those we care about, we need to share laughter when we can. Seeing the humor in a situation relieves some of the tension and provides a break from the pain. Laughing and crying are not that different from one another; each allows a letting go of feelings, expressions of the comic and tragic aspects of life.

IMPACT OF CFIDS ON FAMILIES

Chronic illness disrupts a family's usual patterns and dynamics. All families develop ways of coping with stress over time, but chronic illness is an unexpected and unusual type of stress which lingers and causes continuing disruption. Families that are cohesive, flexible, resourceful, and adaptable will be more success-ful at coping with CFIDS. The following suggestions can help:

Talk about what's happening. Pretending it's not there won't make it go away. Discuss the illness and its effects on the family as a whole and on individual family members. Don't assign blame; discuss the illness as a shared problem. Make sure that all family members have an understanding of the illness, even young children.

Open communication requires that all family members should be allowed to speak for themselves, not for one another, and that each accepts the others' feelings as valid. This means not trying to talk others out of how they feel or expecting them to become optimistic when they're concerned or depressed. Em-pathize with the others' feelings, even when you wish they didn't feel that way. When the PWC says, "I'm scared that I'll never recover," instead of saying, "That's ridiculous—of course you will!", a more empathetic statement would be, "I know this is frightening for you. Not knowing can be very hard." This allows the PWC to feel understood and supported, rather than told how to feel.

Develop as much flexibility as possible in the way the family functions. Brainstorm to seek solutions to new problems. If responsibilities have to be reassigned, make sure each family member is clear about what is expected of them.

In many families one person is unofficially regarded as the caretaker. This may be the person who now has CFIDS. All

family members should assume some of the caretaking responsibilities, rather than regarding them as the responsibility of
only one person. This lessens the burden on any one individual
and teaches valuable skills to the others.

The PWC should be open in discussing his or her limitations and problems rather than covering them up in an attempt
to shield the family from difficulty and pain. However, the
PWC should avoid becoming overly dependent on other family
members, especially young children. Taking on primary support
of a parent is an inappropriate burden for a child.

The family should avoid attempts to overprotect the PWC,
and avoid making assumptions about what the PWC can do or
would like to do. The PWC should be involved whenever
possible in making family plans and given the option of parti-
cipating.

If extended family members, neighbors, or others in the
community are available, they can provide additional support
and perhaps help with the additional responsibilities created by
the illness.

The needs of all family members, not just the PWC, must
be understood and respected. In addition to showing caring for
the ill family member, each must consider personal well-being
a priority.

Children of PWCs often resent the limitations imposed
on their lives by the illness. They may react by becoming
demanding or depressed, by blaming themselves for the illness
or family problems, or by developing behavior problems at school
and/or at home. They may be unaware of the connection between their behavior and their parent's illness and the conse-
quent disruption of stability in their lives. Their reactions and
behaviors should be discussed openly and reassurance offered.
Help in the form of individual or family therapy should be
sought if the problems increase or do not resolve over time. In
any case, it is neither helpful nor healthy to condone or ignore
a child's inappropriate behavior because the parent feels guilty
or incapable of discipline.

Express caring for one another openly through words and
gestures. Touch; hug. Don't assume that the others know you

love them—let them know! Acknowledge their feelings. Express hope. Let all family members know that they are valuable and helpful to the family. Sharing these feelings can create new strength, growth, and closeness.

FOR SINGLE PWCS

Enduring CFIDS as a single person is a mixed bag. You have the privacy and freedom to make your own schedule without taking someone else's needs into account. However, you may also lack the comfort of a primary support person. There's no one else to take up the financial slack, to complain to, to bring you tea and toast. (Remember, however, that some partners of PWCs are unwilling to do these things.) You may be forced to live with parents or grown children, leading to feelings of dependence and perhaps guilt.

If you are dating or seeking a permanent relationship, the issue of what to tell the other person inevitably comes up. It is usually best not to disclose detailed information too soon—but don't keep your illness a secret either. Look for a middle ground between these extremes and you will find the level of disclosure that works best for you. CFIDS adds a difficult dimension to new relationships; some thrive anyway and others don't last. Some people will distance themselves at the mention of CFIDS, usually because of their own fears and prejudices or their unwillingness to become involved with someone who is ill.

Even if a primary relationship is not feasible for you right now, don't isolate yourself. Plan at least minimal activities that involve contact with the outside world, such as trips to the library, a class, or a movie. Interact with others, stay in touch with friends and relatives, as well as other PWCs. It's vital that you have a support system.

WHEN THE PWC IS A CHILD

Children generally require more attention than adults. They should be given information about CFIDS that is appropriate for their age and should be encouraged to ask questions. Don't be afraid to say, "I don't know" if you cannot answer their questions. Try to be reassuring but don't withhold the truth, as this may jeopardize their trust. Ask them about their feelings: Do they feel left out of important activities? Ignored by their peers? Burdensome to the family? Different, not okay? Unable to do "normal" things? They may be able to express their feelings and needs quite clearly, or might require your help to clarify them.

If the child's attendance at school is a problem, look into resources for home instruction. Educate the child's teacher about CFIDS (especially its cognitive effects) and work cooperatively to develop a flexible and appropriate learning plan. If you encounter resistance from the school administration, pursue the matter assertively with the help of your health care providers and a local support group if necessary.

CFIDS may prolong a child's dependence on the family, an especially difficult issue with adolescents. Discuss this problem openly. Allow for as much autonomy in decision-making by the child as possible.

Consider the use of guided imagery (as described in Chapter 11) for self-expression and healing. Children are often more responsive to imagery than adults because they haven't yet acquired adult constraints and are usually open to playing an active role.

Don't neglect other children in the family. If they are resentful about the "privileged" status of the child with CFIDS (fewer responsibilities, more attention), allow them to express their feelings openly but not in a way that is demeaning or blaming of their ill sibling.

Treat the child with CFIDS as normally as possible. Try not to make too many special exceptions. Illness, although genuine, can be used manipulatively. Continue discipline, routines, and family structure as before to whatever degree possible. Be aware of any tendency to "baby" or rescue the child, or to "make up for" the illness with inappropriate favors or privileges. You cannot compensate for the child's losses.

Children, especially teenagers, may attempt to deny health problems, theirs or anyone else's. Let them know gently that denial won't work, that facing illness is painful but they are strong enough to do so and will have the family's support. Then allow them to express their feelings (don't "correct" them) and to grieve. Don't expect their feelings to make sense or to match yours; allow them to experience and accept illness in their own way.

Try to plan fun activities and allow the child to interact with friends as much as possible. Peer relationships are extremely important to kids; don't be insulted if peer activities take precedence over family ones.

Children are very adaptable and are capable of handling hardships and illnesses such as CFIDS amazingly well. Like all of us, they need frequent signs of support and encouragement—only more so.

RELATIONSHIPS IN THE WORKPLACE

If you are able to continue working, there have probably been changes in your attendance record, work hours, and relationships with employer and coemployees. PWCs often wonder what to tell employers and prospective employers about the illness. It's not wise to hide or lie about your illness. In the long run the cover-up may be difficult to sustain, and greater problems may ensue if your health status is discovered later on. If CFIDS does not interfere with your ability to work productively, however, there may be no reason to volunteer health information. There is no universally correct way to handle this situation; it's a matter of your own preference and judgment.

Many employers are quite understanding of the special needs created by CFIDS and even request information about the illness. Others are less tolerant. The work setting and your responsibilities might not offer the flexibility you need right now. If you are unable to meet the requirements of your present job, consider alternatives: switch to a less demanding job, cut back on work hours, do your work at home, or explore disability benefits if necessary.

If you work closely with others, some of your symptoms are likely to become apparent to coworkers. Again, you must decide what and how much to disclose. You may want to give them general information about your illness, especially those with whom you work closely. Explain how CFIDS affects you, including the unpredictable changes in mood and behavior, so they won't misunderstand you. Encourage them to ask questions. Be honest about how you feel. Expect that some coworkers will be understanding and supportive, and some will not.

Discrimination in the workplace has been a problem for many PWCs. The newly adopted Americans with Disabilities Act will be helpful to those who have experienced job-related discrimination.

RELATIONSHIPS WITH FRIENDS

Relationships change in different ways in response to the stresses of CFIDS. Some continue relatively unchanged, some become closer, and some dissolve. New friendships may be sought with both PWCs and "civilians." A mixture provides a balance between the support only other PWCs can provide, and the contact with the outside world and perspectives offered by healthier friends. Different types of friendships have different characteristics. Some revolve around shared interests or activities; others are based on common traits or professions. Some are just for fun—humor, movies, leisure activities. Deeper relationships involve more intimate sharing. Having a variety of friends can reduce boredom and loneliness.

Most PWCs feel a strong, ongoing need to talk with others about their illness and its impact on their lives. Different relationships will tolerate different amounts of focus on your illness. With close friends you can discuss the impact of your present needs on the relationship. In more distant relationships the talk about CFIDS will be more superficial; in-depth discussions could strain relationship boundaries. Even though CFIDS is the main event in your life, you will need to make decisions about how much discussion of the illness is appropriate in each of your relationships.

Your friends will not always know how to respond to your statements about CFIDS. They may think you are exaggerating, and respond with disbelief. Talk about it, tell them what it's like, but don't let CFIDS take over. If their reactions are consistently disappointing, you may need to confront them, or even end the relationship.

The energy crunch and isolative tendencies that often accompany CFIDS make friendships difficult. Not everyone can understand or tolerate our alternating needs for distance and closeness. If you are fortunate, most of your friendships will last, but not all relationships can survive the toll of chronic illness.

ABOUT SUICIDE: SUGGESTIONS FOR FRIENDS AND FAMILY

During times of desperation, most PWCs have considered suicide as the only route for escaping their great emotional pain. Although relatively few follow through with their plans, the incidence of suicide is significantly higher among PWCs than in the general population. Suicidal talk or behavior should always be taken seriously.

Discouraging relapses may lead to the irrational thinking (which seems quite real and logical at the time) that recovery will never take place, life is too painful to endure, no one cares, and no hope exists. Trying to talk a suicidal person out of being pessimistic is usually ineffective, but you can help by listening. Keep communication going. Allow the patient to do most of the talking as you pay careful attention. Be supportive but not unrealistically optimistic, as this would only cause the patient to feel misunderstood. Ask what you can do to help. Stay with the person until you are certain that any danger has passed. If you need to leave for a period of time, ask if the patient needs anything and will feel safe being alone. Suggest resources such as counseling, group therapy, or contact with other PWCs. Once the initial feelings are expressed and you feel the timing is right, help the patient identify reasons to live, to hope. If depression is severe and does not lift and suicide is a possibility, hospitalization may be appropriate.

AN OPEN LETTER FROM
A CFIDS PATIENT TO A FRIEND

Dear Friend,

I know my illness is putting pressure on both of us and is straining our relationship. Don't give up on me! Please try to be patient. I have unpredictable mood swings. Sometimes I'm so depressed I want the whole world to go away and I don't want to talk to anyone. Please don't take it personally. I just need to pull back until I can interact productively again.

Let's talk together about the changes in me and the changes in our relationship. I know you've noticed them and I'd like the opportunity for us to discuss them openly. Please tell me about your life, too, even if I forget to ask. I get very self-absorbed when I feel ill and discouraged, but I still care about you. If I forget to show my caring, please let me know, gently. Your needs matter to me a lot, but sometimes mine get in the way.

I need lots of attention right now, lots of caring. I don't want my needs to overwhelm you but sometimes they overwhelm me. I don't expect you to rescue me, to make me all better, but I hope you're willing to listen while I express needs, emotions, and thoughts. Sometimes I'll need to bounce ideas off you to get some feedback. I'll try to make my needs known; tell me if I'm not being clear or if I'm expecting too much.

There are times I think I can't get through this; please remind me that I'm strong and that I've gotten through so far. Tell me you believe in me.

I feel guilty because right now I don't have much to give. Our relationship is uneven, unbalanced, and I don't feel good about being the one with greater needs. I don't expect to be babied or coddled but I often need a lot of attention and caring. I sometimes feel as if I'm a burden and you're just tolerating me to be nice. I know better; this is my insecurity I'm talking about—not you. I would like to repay you somehow, even though you probably don't expect to be repaid.

Please continue to stay in touch and invite me to do things with the understanding that I may have to respond with "maybe" or "no," wishing I could join you. Try to realize that what seems to you like a minor exertion can be a major effort for me; when I'm not doing well such an effort can deplete my energy resources and may jeopardize my health even further. I miss doing things with you but need to be very careful about my activity level.

I both love and hate it when you tell me I'm looking good. Please don't assume that means I'm feeling good. And when you ask how I am, I'll answer honestly but will try to summarize and not ramble too much or bore you.

I know you can't always be available to me, and I'll try to understand when you have conflicting needs of your own. CFIDS has helped me to realize the importance of feeling cared about. Thank you for being my friend.

An Open Letter from a CFIDS Patient to a Spouse/Partner

Dear "Significant Other,"

Please understand that I am going through a horrible ordeal. My moods and behaviors are unplanned and unpredictable, and I feel horrible about inflicting my illness on you. I know you're affected by my changes, and I wish it were otherwise. I don't want to be ill.

I feel guilty about not being able to shoulder my former responsibilities at work and at home, leaving you to take up the slack. I wish I could do more, or even know in advance what I will be able to do each day. Maybe sometimes you think I'm lazy or just trying to get out of doing something I don't like to do, but that's not it. Sometimes I just can't, and other times I know it would be a mistake to use up all my energy on a minor thing and then have to give up something more important.

I want to know that I can trust you, that you will be available to listen and try to understand. And I'll try to understand that you can't always be available.

At times my feelings are irrational, and I may become angry for no apparent reason. These mood swings are part of my illness. I'll try to keep them under control, but I need you to understand that even when I direct them at you, I'm not blaming you for my illness. I'll try not to use you as a scapegoat for my anger but will sometimes fail. Please don't take my mood swings personally; they're not your fault. If they become too hard to take and you feel ready to explode at me, please tell me so. Maybe one of us can leave the scene if necessary, and we can talk about it later when we're both calmer.

Sometimes I need to talk about these irrational feelings. Just listen, okay? Please don't tell me how to feel or how not to feel. You don't have to "fix" my feelings, and please don't judge them. Just accept and acknowledge them. When you such things as, "CFIDS must be terribly frustrating for you," I feel understood and comforted. But don't tell me you know how I feel. You don't, and you can't; no one can know exactly what this is like for me. And when I cry, don't try to get me to stop. Please let me cry—I'll feel better later.

I know I complain a lot. It helps to relieve tension. If I'm complaining more than you can bear, please tell me so, gently. I probably won't handle it well, but I really do understand that you need to distance yourself from my complaints.

I need to work at making clear requests so that you'll know what I need. It's not your job to mind-read—it's my responsibility to ask for what I want. This is difficult for me; it's easier for me to meet others' needs than to ask others to meet mine.

Don't try to talk me out of my symptoms or remind me that they're not as bad as they could be or not as bad as they were. I know I need to stay hopeful, but if you take an optimistic role when I feel pessimistic, it feels as if you don't understand me or validate my feelings.

I know you don't understand why I'm sick. Neither do I. It's frustrating not to have someone or something to blame, but let's acknowledge our feelings of helplessness to each other.

I don't want you to give up your whole life for me. Please continue to do the things that are important to you. I won't always be able to do them with you, so do them alone. Sometimes I resent not being able to do things and I may even resent your freedom. I'll try to keep a good perspective. If you put your life on hold because of my illness, I'll feel guilty and in time you'll come to resent me. I appreciate your invitations to do things. Your asking lets me know that you still value my company. Please don't assume what I can or can't do; ask, and I'll answer you honestly. I hope you will understand that when I say "no," it's not because I don't want to but because I can't or shouldn't.

I know I'm not the way I used to be. Let's talk about these CFIDS-related changes. I'm trying to learn from my illness, and you can help. We can't pretend that things are the way they were or that they'll ever be the same again. But as we change and grow, let's grow together rather than apart. Let's keep the lines of communication open. When I need to withdraw, I'll try to let you know so you won't take it personally. Please do the same for me. Don't just pull away; explain to me that you need to distance temporarily so I'm less inclined to feel abandoned.

Because we're both experiencing losses, we'll both need to grieve. Some of our grieving will be a solitary process, but some of it will be shared, because we've both lost so much. Let's acknowledge what we've lost by mourning together.

Please don't try to make my decisions for me. If you see me wearing down and think I should rest, please offer your observation, not advice or an order. I need to take care of myself and you can help, but don't try to take over my care. It wouldn't be good for either of us. Your encouragement helps me to do a better job of taking care of myself.

It helps me to have both my difficulties and my strengths acknowledged by you. Tell me you think I'm brave, that I'm fighting hard, that I'm weathering this calamity well. Tell me you still love me. Small tokens help—a flower, a phone call, a card. Tell me you care about me and why you value me. Please touch me; I need hugs now more than ever. Sometimes I may be unable to hear you or I may even push you away when I'm hurting, especially at times when I can't love myself. I'll try not to hurt you, but if I do, please understand that it's not you I'm rejecting, it's me and my illness.

I know our sexual relationship has changed and that we both miss the way it was. I don't know how to explain to you that my lack of energy or sexual interest is a result of my illness and not a rejection of you. I want us to continue to relate physically—to touch, hug, and cuddle. We need to remain close in every way we can.

These are rough times for us. I appreciate the efforts you've made to help me to cope and to be as comfortable as possible. I know I've been difficult to live with. At times you have been too. If we can get through these times together, our relationship will become stronger—something I want very much.

AN OPEN LETTER FROM THE HEALTHY SPOUSE/PARTNER TO THE PWC

Dear PWC Whom I Love,

I know you have overwhelming needs right now due to your illness. I know you have difficulty coping. Please try to see that I'm going through a hard time, too. I almost feel as if I shouldn't have needs, but your illness affects me as well, very deeply. I care about you, and when you hurt and I can't fix it then I hurt too.

I feel helpless, perhaps even more helpless than you do. I wish I knew how to make you better. Sometimes I give you too much advice. It's not always helpful but sometimes I don't know what else to give, and I want to give something. I'll try not to take over your care or tell you what's best for you. I don't want you to be dependent on me any more than you have to be.

Please tell me what you need. I won't repeat your confidences to anyone. Sometimes you hold back and I become frustrated because I don't know what you need. If you ask me to do something specific for you, I have the option of saying "yes" or "no." But you have to ask.

I take what you say seriously, even though some of it doesn't make sense to me. Please take what I say seriously as well, even when I don't make sense to you.

There are times when I just don't understand. You seem crazy, or lazy, or as if you no longer care about *my* needs. I know it isn't true but I can't help my feelings. I guess you sometimes need to feel sorry for yourself. I feel sorry for myself, too, and I'm not even the one who's sick.

Sometimes you dump on me when you're especially tired or grouchy. I understand this in my head, but I still hurt. I feel as if you're blaming me for your illness and expecting me to fix it. I'd do anything I can to help you, but I can't make it go away. Please try not to lash out. If something is really bothering you, let's try to talk about it at a good time.

When I do something that's helpful, please tell me so. I need feedback and acknowledgement from you. I'm doing an awful lot right now. I need to know that what I'm doing is noticed and appreciated.

I love you, but I need other friends and family in my life as well. I hope that my time with them won't cause you to feel left out when you're not feeling well enough to participate. I may become overly involved in work and other activities because of my need for time out. I'm trying to balance our needs, and just as you need to take care of yourself, I need to take care of myself. This is new for both of us. I still need to see friends, exercise, play, and deal with job stresses, family needs, and my own health concerns.

I agree that we should continue to make decisions together, even though I may have to carry them out alone. I'll try not to be a martyr or a dictator. If you see that I'm making too many decisions without your input and you feel left out, please tell me.

Sometimes I think you should do things differently in order to get better. When I ask you to try some special treatment, diet, or positive thinking, it's because I'm trying to help. Sometimes I even get mad at your doctor, thinking that with adequate care you'd get better.

Although I try not to burden you with the way I feel, I don't want to pretend I have no bad feelings about this. I feel afraid, hurt, vulnerable, angry, and sad at times. Sometimes I become angry at you for being sick, although rationally I know it's not your fault.

When you are depressed or stay in bed, staring into space, I feel abandoned. I *know* you're not abandoning me, but I *feel* vulnerable. Sometimes I think this illness has taken over your life, and I'm not very important anymore. Please let me know that I'm still important to you.

Let's try to do some fun things together. I know your energy is limited, but we need some time off from the gloom. Let's figure out what we can do to enjoy each other. Save some of your precious energy for *us*, even if it's just to watch a videotape together and share some popcorn.

We can get through this together. Despite the pain and the struggles, let's not forget how much we mean to each other.

Chapter 14

◆

Conclusion

FOLKSINGER PETE SEEGER told a story many years ago about a king who wanted to have all the world's wisdom condensed into one book. He appointed a wise man to perform this awesome task but refused to read the book when it was presented to him, saying, "Now boil everything in this book down to one page." And when presented with the wisdom of the world in one page, again the king did not read it but asked that it be condensed into one paragraph. When the wise man had done this, the king asked him to condense it into one word. When he returned, the king asked for the one word that held the world's wisdom, and the wise man told the king, "The word is 'maybe.'"

Now that I have spent years treating and interviewing PWCs, and researching and writing about CFIDS, I find that I really have little to offer in the way of definitive, universal conclusions or recommendations. Quite frankly, I feel inadequate writing a book based on maybes—but maybes is all we've got.

We want more. We need answers to our questions, further research funding, more positive attention and treatment from the medical community, a revised illness definition from the CDC, greater recognition and concern from the Social Security Administration, and the knowledge that our plight is being taken seriously by our government, health care providers, and loved ones.

We can provide the impetus for these changes by speaking up; by supporting our local and national support groups (of which there are more than five hundred!); by writing letters to legislators and organizations; and by educating ourselves, our health care providers, and concerned others.

Paul Cheney, M.D., testified about this "monstrous and yet subtle disease" before the Senate Appropriations Subcommittee on Labor, Health and Human Services, and Education in Washington, D.C. on May 8, 1989:

> The most remarkable thing about chronic fatigue syndrome is that the impetus for its recognition as a defined clinical entity has come primarily from patients. If there was ever a grassroots disease, this is it. What clues there are to this disorder lie *presently* in listening carefully to these patients.
>
> The CDC now receives one hundred calls from patients and physicians each week. CFIDS-related calls to the NIAID, an AIDS-dominated institution in Bethesda, Maryland, are outnumbered only by AIDS-related calls. Thousands of social security and private disability claims list CFIDS as the principal cause of disability. Many school systems provide homebound instruction to children with this disorder. This disorder has already or will likely cost this country billions in lost productivity and health costs, and ironically from its most productive segment, the young and middle-aged adult. It could easily dwarf the economic effects of AIDS and sap the nation of its economic vitality (*The CFIDS Chronicle*, Spring 1989).

There are millions of PWCs in the United States alone, and, unfortunately, our number is growing. We are faced with individual and collective struggles. As a group we share concerns regarding CFIDS recognition, health care, and social issues. Individually we struggle with physiological, spiritual, and emotional issues. We survive this ordeal as best we can despite dwindling checkbook balances, bizarre symptoms, and alternating hope and despair.

I have grown during the time I have been ill, and I have learned some things I would never even have thought about had I remained well. I am not pretending to be glad I have

CFIDS; I would just as soon be well and make do with a little less growth. But I don't have that choice, so I've decided to make the best of it in my own way. I hope you will do the same.

Susan Levine, M.D., wrote about CFIDS: "This is a silent illness which . . . robs people of their day to day sanity." Well, this illness can *borrow* my sanity, but it can't *have* it. CFIDS can spur me to examine the meaning of life in general, and of my life in particular, and it can create obstacles in everything from relationships to my ability to think coherently, but it can't take over permanently and it can't destroy my life. Tomorrow I may think differently, but my wish is to have many more hopeful and productive days like today. I can live with that.

Appendix A

◆

R & R:
Research and Resources

The important thing is not to stop questioning.
Albert Einstein

CFIDS research is being conducted at several prestigious institutions and more informally in doctors' offices across the country. Through scientific research in combination with the serendipitous findings that often lead to breakthroughs, researchers may discover the causes, treatments, and ultimately cures for CFIDS. Andrew Lloyd pointed out that studies to date have been physician-based rather than community-based, that is, only those who have been diagnosed and treated by physicians are being studied. Those in the community who have self-diagnosed or undiagnosed CFIDS have not been included, thus potentially altering the true picture (November 1991).

Although several government agencies are now involved in conducting CFIDS research, most research to date has been funded by the private sector through donations of patients and concerned others and in great part due to the fundraising efforts of Drs. Cheney, Elaine DeFreitas, John Martin, and others.

NATIONAL ATTENTION TO CFIDS

Unfortunately, as a nation we have taken an ostrich-like approach to chronic viral and immune dysfunction-related illnesses. Given the magnitude of the problem, relatively little has been done to solve it.

Society's general attitude toward AIDS is a good example. Our deepest fears and prejudices about this lethal, out-of-control illness led to our avoiding the HIV problem until it was a disease of epidemic proportions. Although the problem has existed since at least the late 1970s, little attention was focused on it until two shocking events occurred: the public became aware of AIDS in the heterosexual, non-drug-using population, and Rock Hudson, a national idol, died of it. Then it got real for us. By that time it had spread dramatically and thousands of people had died, but research funding was still woefully inadequate. The disease just wasn't pleasant or convenient to deal with. We boast a huge federal budget, national research institutes, state-of-the-art health care resources, outstanding media involvement and coverage of health issues, and a humanitarian philosophy. But we turn a deaf ear to the cries of those afflicted with chronic immune-related illnesses. The bureaucracy is too busy. Politics and finances are more important than human lives.

The approach initially taken by the press to CFIDS was disappointing. All we read was about the crazy and lazy people with an imaginary new yuppie illness, an excuse to cop out. CFIDS was treated like a second-class illness seen in those unable to cope productively with life, a first cousin to hypochondria.

The government's reaction to the CFIDS problem has been as underwhelming as its response to the AIDS epidemic. It's easy to ignore an illness that's invisible, that doesn't kill people or even make them look sick. Research funding remains inadequate. They have taken a few stabs here and there, waiting for the problem to go away. It hasn't. Several government health agencies that fall under the auspices of the United States Public Health Service have played a role in the study of CFIDS: the National Institutes of Health (NIH), Centers for Disease Control (CDC), National Institute of Allergy and Infectious Diseases (NIAID), National Cancer Institute (NCI), National Center for Research Resources (NCRR), National Institute of Neurological Disorders and Stroke (NINDS), National Institute of Child Health and Human Development (NICHD), and National Institute of Arthritis, Musculoskeletal and Skin Diseases (NIAMS). Their efforts to date have been inadequate.

The NIH has no staff assigned to CFIDS on a full-time basis. The NIH recently held an "open" meeting about CFIDS that was not well publicized, ostensibly to consider an update of the diagnostic criteria. Although some CFIDS experts were invited to this meeting, they were not listened to, and many important researchers and clinicians were not invited at all. Numerous studies are underway at various branches of the NIH, but the study of CFIDS remains grossly underfunded.

The current CDC surveillance effort in four cities (Atlanta, Reno, Grand Rapids, and Wichita—none of them "hot spots") to determine the number of Americans afflicted with CFS/CFIDS is a start, and preliminary results have been published. The CDC has found many more cases of CFIDS than originally estimated. Although important findings will result from this study, it does nothing to meet the current needs of PWCs. The study will be expanded to include children, new sites, and investigations of new outbreaks. Additional CDC personnel are needed to respond to communications from patients and health care providers, and to study possible etiologic agents, virus reactivation, various aspects of immune functioning, laboratory and exposure data, and common exposure factors. A Public Health Service CFS Interagency Committee has been instituted to improve communication between federal health agencies (including the Food and Drug Administration and the National Institutes of Health) and between the CDC and researchers in the private sector. Walter Gunn, Ph.D., as the chief investigator for CFS studies at the CDC has played an active role in helping to solve the CFIDS puzzle and has been responsible for recent progress made by the CDC. He has interacted with other government officials and agencies, made numerous presentations about CFIDS nationally, and discussed CFIDS on radio and television.

NIAID has been conducting ongoing research regarding CFIDS, including viral involvement, prevalence, treatment, and immunological studies. Steven Straus, M.D., head of the Medical Virology section, has been widely criticized for his insistence on characterizing CFIDS as a psychiatric illness, regarding CFIDS in a patronizing and demeaning way. NIAID publishes an "Update" that summarizes current knowledge about CFIDS. Dr. Ann Schluederberg, a virology program officer at NIAID, stressed NIAID's continued interest in CFIDS by offering research grants, generating publications and holding workshops (1988). Again, government rhetoric has led us to believe that CFIDS is being studied aggressively, but NIAID has been criticized by CFIDS researchers for lack of follow-through, indicating that CFIDS is not being taken seriously enough. Dennis Jackson, Ph.D., noted in his "Media Watch" column in The CFIDS Chronicle that NIAID was "conspicuous by its absence" in the well-known comprehensive *Newsweek* CFIDS article, and that NIAID and Straus would be "relegated to the deserved oblivion they will receive when the history of this severe, enigmatic disease is recorded in medical textbooks."

Three extramural research centers will be funded by NIAID to conduct multidisciplinary CFIDS studies. The centers will be located in Boston, Denver, and Newark, New Jersey. Goals are establishment of a standardized way to evaluate CFS patients, including diagnostic markers; comparison of PWCs with healthy individuals and those with multiple sclerosis, depression, allergies, fibromyalgia, and rheumatoid arthritis; and abnormalities in genes, virus production, cell function, and organ systems. These efforts are strongly needed but the centers are likely to be underfunded with an allocation of 1.2 million dollars for the first year for all three centers. The National Cancer Institute, National Institute of Arthritis, Musculoskeletal and Skin Diseases, and the Social Security Administration all claim to be interested in the study and dissemination of information regarding CFIDS. However, their degrees of involvement remain to be seen. We need fewer double messages from these institutions and more action.

Strong CFIDS advocacy efforts have been made by such lobbyists as R. Barry Sleight (CFIDS advocate in Washington, DC), Theodore W. Van Zelst (cofounder of Minann, Inc.), and most recently Roy Snoeyenbos. Sleight has retired from CFIDS advocacy and will be missed. CACTUS (CFIDS Action Campaign for the United States) has hired a professional lobbyist, Tom Sheridan, to take his place. Our advocates have been successful in attracting national attention and funding. Although the movement has been slow to get off the ground, it seems that CFIDS is finally beginning to become something of a national priority. Research is being done in other countries as well, notably Canada, England, Germany, Australia, and New Zealand.

In the United States, CFIDS is being studied at such research centers as Duke University, the National Jewish Center for Immunology and Respiratory Medicine in Colorado, the Cheney Clinic in North Carolina, Children's Hospital in Philadelphia, Stanford University, Harvard, University of Massachusetts, Mount Sinai Hospital in New York, the University of North Carolina, and the Wistar Institute. However, inadequate government funding for large-scale research means that much of the available information about CFIDS treatment has come from informal studies done by individual doctors. A number of dedicated physicians have conducted unpaid private research, at considerable expense. Not many can afford to do this, and none can continue indefinitely. Interdisciplinary CFIDS research is vital; individual researchers are handicapped by being isolated from one another and having to network on their own.

Outstanding among the exceptional CFIDS practitioners/researchers are Drs. David Bell (NY), Paul Cheney (NC), Jay Goldstein (CA), Byron Hyde (Canada), James Jones (CO), Anthony Komaroff (MA), and Daniel Peterson (NV). They share a significant trait: all of these physicians have taken CFIDS seriously over the years and have been outspoken even to the point of incurring the wrath of unbelieving and unconcerned medical colleagues. They and other concerned, caring physicians have stood by us, treated us, and defended us (which shouldn't have been necessary in the first place!) and we are most grateful to all of them.

A high level of awareness and a strong commitment to research must be made by the federal government, researchers, physicians, patients, and the public. Paul Cheney, M.D., and others have described some of the obstacles to be overcome in future research: lack of a consensus over case definition, political divisions in research centers and national patient groups, poorly constructed research studies, lack of consistent databases and case definitions which would allow patients to be followed over time, the need for analyses of various subpopulations of patients to establish whether all are suffering from the same illness, need for a multidisciplinary approach, and coordination of efforts between CFIDS research and that involving other possibly related illnesses.

To date we have been penny-wise and pound-foolish by drastically underfunding CFIDS research as the disease takes a huge financial toll in terms of disability benefits, medical expenses, and the lost productivity of PWCs, a sizeable segment of our workforce. CFIDS/immune/virological research must become national and international priorities. Outbreaks of CFIDS and similar illnesses in the past have been largely ignored and forgotten. Such disasters must not reoccur.

PWCs can help promote "the cause" by writing to legislators, stressing the need for CFIDS research funding (in the public and private sectors) and Social Security Administration reform regarding disability benefits for PWCs. Letter writing can have a significant impact on government attention to CFIDS. In addition to the senators and representatives from individual states, numerous government committees must be urged to promote CFIDS efforts; see the Spring/Summer 1990 *CFIDS Chronicle* or your local newsletter for lists. Consider an individual project of collecting and presenting this information to local support groups, along with a sample letter containing relevant information and specific requests for funding.

CONFERENCES

A number of CFIDS conferences and conventions have been held in the United States and abroad. These conferences have been sponsored by national and state CFIDS organizations, individual researchers and research institutions, and government agencies. Some have been research-oriented and some patient-oriented, others have been a combination of both. The primary goal of such meetings has been to share findings and theories from a number of disciplines, including allergy/immunology, neurology, psychology/psychiatry, and environmental medicine. A small number of CFIDS fundraisers have been held as well.

ASSOCIATIONS AND ORGANIZATIONS

Because attention to CFIDS has resulted largely from a grass-roots patient effort, national and local organizations have played a vital role in advocacy and dissemination of information. Several national organizations have been working diligently to promote involvement at all levels. They have been inundated with requests for information about CFIDS. Cooperative work among these organizations would help us to consolidate our efforts and have a greater impact politically.

Contributions to our national, regional, and local organizations are vital to their survival. These groups serve the needs of CFIDS patients by disseminating information regarding possible causes, treatment, coping, support, and reports about legislative advocacy and lobbying efforts. They are our lifeline.

National associations

Membership, newsletters (current and past issues), and other printed information (including local support group contacts, symptom checklists, and reprints of articles from medical journals and the popular press) are available from:

> The CFIDS Association, Inc.
> P.O. Box 220398
> Charlotte, NC 28222-0398   Tel. (704) 362-2343

This organization publishes *The CFIDS Chronicle*, an excellent source of information regarding CFIDS research, current theories, advocacy, and coping suggestions. In addition, the CFIDS Association maintains a Physician's Honor Roll for each state—a list of patient-recommended physicians and other professionals. Literature is available by order, including back issues. Research funding, advocacy, and patient information are major priorities.

For membership information and basic information about CFIDS, call voice mail at The CFIDS Association, Charlotte, NC:

(800) 44-CFIDS   (800-442-3437)

For information on various topics presented by expert clinicians and researchers (main menu includes overview of CFIDS, CFIDS Association, treatment, diagnosis, research updates, CACTUS, CFIDS-related health issues, and CFIDS in children), call

(900) 988-CFID   (900-988-2343)

Charges apply for the second number and begin after the first ten seconds of the recorded message. The proceeds cover the cost of the two telephone lines with the balance going to CFIDS research/advocacy.

Other national organizations providing information, advocacy, or support include:

CFIDS Foundation
965 Mission Street, Suite 425
San Francisco, CA 94103   Tel. (415) 882-9986
They provide literature (including treatment bulletins), telephone counseling, referrals, training, research funding, and advocacy.

Fibromyalgia Network
7001 Schoolhouse Lane
Bakersfield, CA 93309   Tel. (805) 833-8387
They publish quarterly issues of "Fibromyalgia Network"

National Chronic Fatigue Syndrome Association
3521 Broadway, Suite 222
Kansas City, MO 64111   Tel. (816) 931-4777
This association publishes the *Heart of America Newsletter* containing CFIDS articles and patient resource information.

Also available are CFIDS information packets, brochures, audio-
and videotapes, and CFIDS book reviews.

San Francisco CFIDS Task Force
3543 18th Street, #20
San Francisco, CA 94110   Tel. (415) 525-6415
They provide literature, advocacy, support. This organization networks widely with CFIDS groups and PWCs nationwide.

CFIDS Foundation
965 Mission Street, Suite 425
San Francisco, CA 94103   Tel. (415) 882-9986
They provide literature (including treatment bulletins),
telephone counseling, referrals, training, research funding, and
advocacy.

CFS Research Foundation
P.O. Box 6747, Cherry Creek
Denver, CO 80206
They do fundraising for CFIDS research.

Minann, Inc.
P.O. Box 582
Glenview, IL 60025
This private organization promotes CFIDS research and
advocacy.

NORD: National Organization for Rare Disorders, Inc.
P.O. Box 8923
New Fairfield, CT 06812   Tel. (203) 746-6518
They provide information about various illnesses includ-
ing CFIDS.

Buyers' club

CFIDS Buyers' Club
1187 Coast Village Road, #1-280
Santa Barbara, CA 93108   Tel. (800) 366-6056
The Buyer's Club, founded by Rich Carson, offers dis-
counted nutritional supplements and donates a portion of profits
to CFIDS research. A complimentary catalog is available.

Consumer resources

Fraudulent health products may be reported to your state attorney general's office and/or:

The Food and Drug Administration
Consumer Affairs and Information
5600 Fishers Lane
HFC-110
Rockville, MD 20857   Tel. (301) 443-3170

If you have questions about specific health products, send a business-size, self-addressed, stamped envelope and $1 to:

Consumer Health Research Institute
3521 Broadway
Kansas City, MO 64111   (800) 753-8850

If you believe you have been harmed by a quack remedy, write to:

National Council Against Health Fraud
Victim Redress Taskforce
P.O. Box 33008
Kansas City, MO 64114

If mail fraud was involved in your purchase of such products, write:

The U.S. Postal Service
Chief Postal Inspector
475 L'Enfant Plaza
Washington, DC 20260

Government agencies & publications

Information packets are available from the NIH, CDC, and NIAID. Write to the addresses below:

Clinical Center Communications
National Institutes of Health
9000 Rockville Pike
Building 10, Room 1C255
Bethesda, MD 20892   Tel. (301) 496-5717

Their booklet is informative but very basic and contains inaccuracies.

Centers for Disease Control
Division of Viral Diseases; Mail Stop A32
1600 Clifton Road, NE
Atlanta, GA 30333   Tel. (404) 639-1338
Recorded message at (404) 332-4555 (CFS is #7).

National Institute of Allergy and Infectious Diseases
National Institutes of Health
Office of Communications
Building 31, Room 7A32
Bethesda, MD 20892   Tel. (301) 496-5717

The Consumer Information Catalog is a pamphlet listing booklets and fact sheets on a wide variety of topics including Social Security, federal programs, food and nutrition, and health (drugs and health aids, medical problems, and mental health). Materials are free or inexpensive. This catalog may be ordered at no charge from:
Consumer Information Center-2A
P.O. Box 100
Pueblo, CO 81002

A *Summary of Existing Legislation Affecting Persons with Disabilities* and Social Security information may be ordered from:
Superintendent of Documents
U.S. Government Printing Office
Washington, DC 20402

(*Note:* The recently passed Americans with Disabilities Act addresses the requirement that employers make "reasonable accommodations" for disabled employees. Potential implications for the rights of disabled PWCs are encouraging.)

FINANCIAL AID

Information regarding resources for the disabled may be obtained from:

Clearinghouse on Disability Information
U.S. Department of Education
Room 3132 Switzer Building
Washington, DC 20202-2524

For Social Security Disability Benefits information:
Government Entitlement Services
24472 North Western Highway, Suite 200
Southfield, MI 48075   Tel. (800) 678-2887

The National Health Law Program offers services to low-income persons with health care legal problems. Write to:
National Health Law Program, Inc.
2639 S. La Cienega Boulevard
Los Angeles, CA 90034   Tel. (213) 204-6010

National Health Law Program, Inc.
2025 M Street, NW, Suite 400
Washington, DC 20036   Tel. (202) 887-5310

For the name of a local attorney for matters regarding SSDI (disability benefits) or SSI (supplemental income for those not entitled to SSDI), contact your local or national CFIDS support group or:
NOSSCR: National Organization of Social Security
    Claimants' Representatives
19 East Central Avenue
Pearl River, NY 10965
Tel. (800) 431-2804   (914) 735-8812

Books and publications regarding financial aid

Bell, D. (1991) in *The disease of a thousand names*: Disability and its Measurement (chapter) and CFIDS Disability Scale (Appendix II). Pollard Publications, Box 180, Lyndonville, NY 14098.

Brooks, B. & Smith, N. (1988) in *CFIDS: An owner's manual*: Financial aid (chapter). BBNS, Box 6456, Silver Spring, MD 20906.

Casanova, K. (Disability Chairman of The Mass. CFIDS Association). Request the book on applying for Social Security disability. The Mass. CFIDS Association, 808 Main Street, Waltham, MA 02154.

The CFIDS Chronicle: Riding the ox home: A PWC's guide through the social security disability claims process (D.P. Sindicich; Spring/Summer 1990); Sample guide for disability report (Summer/Fall 1989); Your right to disability: persistence pays off (M. Sasser & C. Freese; November/December 1988). Available from the CFIDS Foundation, Inc. Charlotte, NC (address under Organizations).

Imperati, S. & Pearson, J. (1988). *CFIDS social security disability handbook*. Available from CFIDS Association of Charlotte or CFIDS International (addresses under Organizations) and some local support groups.

Ross, J. *Social security benefits: how to get them, how to keep them*. Available from some local support groups or Ross Publishing, 188 Forrester Rd, Slippery Rock, PA 16057.

Smith, D.M. *Disability Workbook for Social Security Applicants*. Available from The CFIDS Association, Inc. of Charlotte, NC.

U.S. Department of Health and Human Services. Understanding Social Security; Supplemental Security Income; Disability; Benefits for Children; Working While Disabled—How Social Security Can Help; The Appeals Process; Medicare (names of individual booklets and fact sheets). Order from Social Security Administration, Baltimore, MD 21235.

These publications offer information and advice about the complicated and confusing process of applying for Social Security (SS) benefits. They cover eligibility requirements, the application process, criteria for selection of an attorney, suggestions for documentation of disability, and tips for maximizing your chances of success. If you are considering applying for SS benefits, be prepared; read some of the above publications and consider consulting an attorney experienced in handling SS cases. Information is also available from national and local support groups.

Other financial resources available in addition to Social Security:

- ✦ Medicare: medical insurance available after two years of disabling illness
- ✦ Medicaid or other state programs: medical services for low-income individuals and families
- ✦ Disability insurance coverage through an employer
- ✦ Supplemental Security Income (SSI), available for those not eligible for Social Security (e.g., those who have not been working prior to onset of illness). Information is available through local Social Security offices
- ✦ State or county aid may be available for housing for low income/disabled, through Housing and Urban Development (HUD). See the government pages of your telephone book for local offices.
- ✦ For other state or county support check with Social Services Department, Department of Economic Security, or city and county information and referral services. Services include food stamps, vocational training, and general welfare.
- ✦ Listings of local resources can also be obtained from:

  Independent Living Centers (300 centers located in all 50 states)—(704) 375-3977.

  National Council on Independent Living—(312) 226-1006.

MEDICAL INSURANCE

Resources for obtaining health insurance include the following:

Employer-sponsored plans Be sure to be familiar with your policy-covered expenses, deductible, coverage for experimental medications, and procedures. Find out if pre-certification is required and in what situations. If you are disabled, you may continue your insurance coverage for a specified period of time through a program called COBRA; you will be financially responsible for paying premiums. Information regarding coverage, including COBRA, should be available from individual employers; large companies have human resource or benefit offices. If you have checked with them and believe you have been given vague or erroneous information, ask to see your policy or benefits booklet. The policy may be detailed and difficult to read but contains the most accurate information regarding coverage.

Individual insurance coverage   You will need to shop around for this both in terms of prices and preexisting conditions. This type of coverage is expensive and difficult for PWCs to qualify for. Currently many insurance companies are in financial trouble and some have gone under. Consider an insurer's track record, especially length of time in business, before purchasing a policy. Information is available from independent insurance agents or representatives of each insurance company.

Medicare   For those not yet of retirement age, Medicare coverage is automatic 24 months after the effective date of Social Security Disability.

Organization group plans   Professional and other organizations may offer insurance plans. However, such organizations may change insurance companies or make changes in the policies while they are in force. The cost is generally less than individual coverage, but individuals still have to qualify for coverage. For information, contact any organizations of which you are a member.

State insurance   The availability, cost and qualifying specifications vary from state to state. For information, call the appropriate state office which should be listed in the government pages of the telephone book.

RESOURCES FOR INDIVIDUAL CFIDS SYMPTOMS

Allergy/immunology/environmental medicine

American Academy for Environmental Medicine
Box 16106
Denver, CO 80216   Tel. (303) 622-9755

Asthma and Allergy Foundation of America
1717 Massachusetts Ave. NW, Suite 305
Washington, DC 20036   Tel. (202) 265-0265

Anxiety, stress and illness

Many hospitals and clinics offer outpatient programs for stress management. Consult your physician, hospital, local or national CFIDS association. The following books are also recommended:

Benson, H. (1976). *The relaxation response.* New York: Avon.

Borysenko, J. (1987). *Minding the body, mending the mind.* Reading, MA: Addison-Wesley.

Pelletier, K. R. (1977). *Mind as healer, mind as slayer.* New York: Dell.

Selye, H. (1974). *Stress without distress.* New York: Signet.

Shealy, C. N. (1979). *90 days to self-health.* New York: Bantam.

Balance disorders

Dizziness and Balance Disorders Association of America
1015 N.W. 22nd Avenue
Portland, OR 97210
Tel. (503) 229-7348;   (800) 227-5726
Publications, newsletter, coping and treatment suggestions.

Levinson, H. L. (1986). *Phobia free.* New York: M. Evans.

Watson, M. A., & Sinclair, H. (1986). *Balancing act: For people with dizziness and balance disorders.* Portland, OR: Good Samaritan Hospital & Medical Center.

Bladder problems

Gillespie, L. (1986). *You don't have to live with cystitis*. New York: Rawson Associates.

Candidiasis

Crook, W. G. (1986). *The yeast connection: A medical breakthrough*. New York: Random House.

Senerchia, D. (1990). *The Silent Menace*. San Francisco: Strawberry Hill.

Trowbridge, J. P. & Walker, M. (1986). *The yeast syndrome*. New York: Bantam.

Chronic pain

Many hospitals and clinics have outpatient programs for pain management. Contact your physician, hospital, or support group for a referral.

Endometriosis

Women with CFIDS and endometriosis are asked to submit their names and addresses for inclusion in a data bank, whose purpose is to encourage research into the suspected links between these two illnesses. For a release form and further information:

The Endo/CFIDS Data Project
P.O. Box 501
Hillsborough, NC 27278

Ballweg, M. L. & The Endometriosis Association. (1987) *Overcoming Endometriosis*. Chicago, IL: Congdon & Weed, Inc.

Sjögren's Syndrome

Sjögren's Syndrome Foundation, Inc.
29 Gateway Drive
Great Neck, NY 11021
Provides information and newsletter regarding Sjögren's

syndrome. Sjögren's Syndrome may be more prevalent in the CFIDS population, but no studies have been done to confirm this.

Visual impairment

Consult your physician or the yellow pages to locate a low vision clinic in your area. Optical aids and coping/compensation techniques are available. Additionally, the Library of Congress provides Talking Books through the National Library Service for the blind and those with physical disabilities. Applications to qualify for such services are handled at the state level, and assistance is available for those who are visually impaired or who have hand weakness that makes it impossible to hold books.

National Library Service for the Blind and Physically Handicapped (Library of Congress): (202) 287-5100.

FURTHER READING

The list of books and resources below is not intended as an endorsement. These are sources of information for PWCs and their significant others. It is vital that the patient work with credentialed, experienced health care personnel in making decisions regarding treatment.

Most CFIDS support groups maintain libraries from which patients may borrow various materials, including books, audiotapes, videotapes, and reprints of medical journal and popular press articles. Public libraries often maintain CFIDS information files as well as CFIDS-related books. The psychology and self-help sections of bookstores are generally well stocked with books that may be helpful to CFIDS patients who wish to use "down time" as an opportunity to learn and grow. Additional resources are listed in the Bibliography.

Medical journal articles about CFIDS

Many CFIDS articles which have appeared in medical journals are available by order from The CFIDS Association, Inc., of

Charlotte, NC and The National Chronic Fatigue Syndrome Association, Kansas City, MO (addresses above). The newsletters published by these and other CFIDS organizations often contain summaries, excerpts, and critiques of the most important articles emerging from current research and practice.

Books about CFIDS

Bell, D. (1991). *The disease of a thousand names: CFIDS*. Pollard Publications, P.O. Box 180, Lyndonville, NY 14098.
   A somewhat technical yet readable book with emphasis on epidemiology, symptomatology, cause, and treatment.

Berne, K. (1990). *CFIDS Lite: chronic fatigue immune dysfunction syndrome with 1/3 the Seriousness*. Available from BHB communications, 761 E. University #F, Mesa, AZ 85203; $12.00 including shipping and handling.
   A humorous look at CFIDS: cartoons, jokes, limericks, etc.

Bolles, E. B. (1990). *Learning to live with chronic fatigue syndrome*. New York: Dell.
   A very superficial and quite inaccurate examination of CFS.

Brooks, B., & Smith, N. (1988). *CFIDS: An owner's manual*. BBNS, P.O. Box 6456, Silver Spring, MD 20906.
   Coping support and suggestions for PWCs.

Conant, S. (1990). *Living with Chronic Fatigue*. Texas: Taylor.
   A well-written book that addresses coping issues.

Feiden, K. (1990). *Hope and help for chronic fatigue syndrome*. New York: Prentice Hall.
   A comprehensive book and well-written book.

Fisher, G. C. (1989). *Chronic fatigue syndrome: A victim's guide to understanding, treating, and coping with this debilitating illness*. New York: Warner.
   A revised and updated version of Fisher's previous book, *Waiting to live*; a somewhat outdated but comprehensive view of the author's experience with CFIDS, along with general information.

Goldstein, J. (1990). *Chronic fatigue syndrome: The struggle for health*. CFS Institute, 436 N. Roxbury Drive, #110, Beverly Hills, CA 90210.

Excellent guide for CFIDS diagnosis and treatment. May be too technical for some PWCs but helpful to physicians.

Jeffreys, T. (1982). *The mile-high staircase*. Auckland: Hodder and Stoughton. Order from Waiake Wordsmiths, P.O. Box 35-429, Browns Bay, Auckland 10, New Zealand; $20.00 surface or $25.00 air mail, payable to A. J. Church.

A personal account of the author's experience with ME (CFIDS)—the first book published on this subject. Interesting and well written.

Stoff, J. A., and Pellegrino, C. R. (1988). *Chronic Fatigue Syndrome: The hidden epidemic*. New York: Random House.

An overly simplistic and misleading view of CFIDS with very controversial treatment suggestions and information. Not recommended.

Wood, T. (1990). *Life in the slow lane*. Woodshed Press, 605 Vantrease Road, Madison, WI 37115.

A personal account of a life slowed down by CFS with emphasis on changed family roles, self-image and coping.

Coping with chronic illness

Lewis, K. S. (1985). *Successful living with chronic illness*. Wayne, NJ: Avery.

Pitzele, S. K. (1986). *We are not alone: learning to live with chronic illness*. New York: Workman.

Register, C. (1987). *Living with chronic illness: Days of patience and passion*. New York: Free Press.

Stearns, A. K. (1984). *Living through personal crisis*. Chicago: Thomas More Press.

Healing and wellness

Borysenko, J. (1990). *Guilt is the teacher, love is the lesson*. New York: Warner.

Borysenko, J. (1987). *Minding the body, mending the mind*. Reading, MA: Addison-Wesley.

Cousins, N. (1989). *Head first*. New York: Dutton.

Cousins, N. (1983). *The healing heart*. New York: Norton.

Cousins, N. (1979). *Anatomy of an illness as perceived by the patient*. New York: Norton.

Locke, S., & Colligan, D. (1986). *The healer within: The new medicine of mind and body*. New York: New American Library.

Matthews-Simonton, S., Simonton, O. C., & Creighton, J. L. (1980). *Getting well again*. New York: Bantam.

Mizel, S. B. & Jaret, P. (1986). *The human immune system: The new frontier in medicine*. New York: Simon & Schuster.

Siegel, B. S. (1986). *Love, medicine and miracles*. New York: Harper & Row.

Weil, A. (1988, rev. ed.). *Health and healing*. Boston: Houghton Mifflin.

For PWCs and their families

Simonton, S. M. (1985). *The healing family*. New York: Bantam Books.

Strong, M. (1988). *Mainstay: For the well spouse of the chronically ill*. Boston: Little, Brown.

Medical care

Berger, S. M. (1988). *What your doctor didn't learn in medical school . . . and what you can do about it*. New York: Morrow.

Inlander, C. B., Levin, L. S., & Weiner, E. (1988). *Medicine on trial*. New York: Prentice Hall.

Robin, E. D. (1984). *Matters of life and death: Risks versus benefits of medical care.* New York: W.H. Freeman.

Weil, A. (1988, rev. ed.). *Health and Healing.* Boston: Houghton Mifflin.

CFIDS *audiotapes*

CFIDS Audiotape. Side 1: definition, diagnosis, coping suggestions, and sources of further information. Side 2: relaxation/stress reduction/healing exercise.

Produced and narrated by Katrina Berne, Ph.D. Order from: BHB Communications, 761 E. University, #F, Mesa, AZ 85203; $10.00 including shipping and handling

Other audiotapes on specific CFIDS-related topics are available from national and local CFIDS associations.

Appendix B

◆

Forming a CFIDS Support Group

Having served as a facilitator, speaker, and consultant for several CFIDS support groups, I would like to share my suggestions for forming and facilitating such groups. I am referring here to smaller, support-oriented, self-help groups whose primarily goals are sharing, mutual support, and generating ideas for managing the illness (as opposed to larger, information-oriented groups at the city or state levels).

An initial organizational meeting can bring interested parties together for the purpose of decision making. To find PWCs in your area to form a group, contact the nearest CFIDS Support/Information group in your area. Your organizational meeting date may be publicized in their newsletter, in flyers, and through a press release to the media. To send out a press release, consult the yellow pages for names of local newspapers and other periodicals, and mail them a press release following the guidelines below. Generally they will be happy to publicize your meeting at no cost and in some cases will even contact you for further information so they can write an article about CFIDS and your group. It is wise to send new press releases periodically, e.g., every few months, to keep the public informed and your group membership strong.

PRESS RELEASE

Purpose of meeting: Support for persons with Chronic Fatigue Immune Dysfunction Syndrome

Date of meeting: _____

Time: _____

Location: _____

Cost: Free (even if there will be a charge for members later on, there is usually no fee for the first meeting.)

Open to all Persons with CFIDS

For further information: Contact _____
  (organizer's name and telephone number)

(*Note:* Enclose a brief description of CFIDS.)

At the initial meeting, the following issues need to be addressed:

Who will lead the group? (a peer? a counselor or
  psychologist? In the latter case, there will generally
  be a charge.) Options: the group leader may be a
  PWC, may alternate between PWCs, or be a
  therapist or other professional—or the group may
  start off being led by a therapist and become
  self-sustained at some point.
Where and when will the group meet?
How long will each meeting last? (90-minute meetings
  are suggested.)
What will be the group's goals?
Will there be invited speakers or consultants? If there is
  a charge, how much will each member contribute?
Will there be a fee for the group? (Costs may include
  room use, mailing, telephone, speakers, refreshments.)
Group size: maximum number of participants. (Six to
  twelve people is a good group size, allowing for
  diverse input but maintaining comfort and intimacy.)

Will significant others be included? At every meeting or at specified meetings (e.g., every fourth meeting)?

Will a telephone tree be developed to keep members informed of new information or meeting changes? Although difficult to develop, a telephone tree saves one individual having to make all the calls; advisable if the group is large.

Once the first meeting gets underway, the issue of confidentiality should be discussed. Those present will need to agree not to discuss the disclosures of others outside the group setting.

A suggested agenda for support group meetings would include:

Introductions: An opportunity for the group leader and each PWC to offer a brief biographical sketch and medical history, as well as hopes and expectations regarding the group and specific areas of concern.

Information: It is helpful to provide members with general CFIDS information, including data regarding larger local groups, national organizations, and a bibliography. Community resource lists should be available.

Topics of common interest: Such topics include discussions of the content areas listed and others, according to the needs of the group.

TOPICS FOR DISCUSSION

General information/discussion about CFIDS
— Onset
— Symptoms (general or physical, emotional, neurological)
— Diagnosis
— The exacerbation/remission cycle
— Relapse "triggers" and techniques for minimizing them

Emotional effects of CFIDS
— Common feelings among PWCs
— Life changes brought about by CFIDS
— Changes in self-concept and self-esteem
— Individual feelings of group members
— Anxiety
— Depression
— Mood swings, irritability, "overreaction"
— Losses and stages of grieving (denial, bargaining, anger, depression, acceptance)
— Coping with emotions
— Expression of feelings
— Learning not to judge feelings

Medical care
— Appropriate medical resources
— Dealing assertively with doctors and other medical personnel
— Avoiding dangerous "fad" treatments
— Emotions regarding medical care (especially fears)

Lifestyle management
— Advantages of learning to manage time and cut back on activities
— Moderation and self-pacing
— Seeking a balance between self-care and responsibilities

Life philosophy
— Shifting the focus to the here and now
— Lessons learned from/during the illness
— Healthy optimism (versus false optimism and versus pessimism)

CFIDS and relationships
— Effects of CFIDS on relationships
— Coping with CFIDS in relationships
— Partners
— Friends
— Family members
— People in the workplace
— Problem-solving in relationships

Advocacy
— Letter-writing to local, state and national
   representa-tives regarding funding for CFIDS research
   (work with your local or national CFIDS support
   group)
— Fund raising for advocacy and research. Local public
   health agencies or support groups for other illnesses
   may become involved in this effort at your request
   (See Feiden's *Hope and Help for Chronic Fatigue
   Syndrome*, pp. 176–179)

Individual CFIDS-related problems
— Brainstorming solution possibilities
— Offering support and affirmation

Some groups require attendance at all meetings regardless
of how ill an individual may feel. Others operate on a "drop-in"
basis: PWCs may attend as they feel the need. Some groups
specify a number of sessions or months the group will meet and
others keep it open-ended, continuing for as long as the demand
exists. If the group does disband, referral of group members to
other support groups is helpful.

Groups differ in terms of "group personality"—a product
of the chemistry between its members. If you have any concerns about the group—for example, an individual who dominates most discussions, or someone presenting what you believe
to be misinformation about CFIDS—it is best to address these
issues immediately and diplomatically in the group session.

Keep the focus of the group open and realistically positive.
Avoid getting stuck in an "ain't it awful" rut in which the tone
of the group is dominated by complaints and hopelessness. If a
group member seems unusually emotionally upset or is not
receiving necessary medical care, make appropriate referrals.

Resource articles:

Pioneering your own support strategies: Carleen Malone, *The
CFIDS Chronicle*, Summer/Fall 1989, pp. 92–97.

The view from the other side of the couch: Linda Miller
Iger, same issue, pp. 102–104.

Appendix C

$$\blacklozenge$$

Publishing a
CFIDS Newsletter

Many local groups publish CFIDS newsletters. Based on many
I have read and reviewed, I offer the following suggestions.

CONTENTS

General CFIDS information

Local and national events regarding CFIDS and chronic
    illness, including date, time, location, speaker, cost

Editorial comment and letters to the editor

Articles contributed by editorial staff and by individual
    PWCs that are of general interest to those with CFIDS
    (e.g., emotional issues, coping, medical treatment,
    information for significant others, anecdotes, suggestions)

A disclaimer stating that the newsletter is intended to
    offer information and support but not to replace
    medical advice or treatment (A local attorney may
    be willing to help you with proper wording)

Summaries of meetings, conventions, and symposia

Reviews and summaries of articles in medical literature
    and other periodicals, books, audiotapes,
    pamphlets—including ordering information

Referral list of local professionals (physicians, attorneys, psychologists/psychiatrists/counselors) recommended by PWCs (contact these professionals first to see if they would like to be placed on the referral list)

Helpline: a telephone number to call for CFIDS support and information, the hours this line is operated, and by whom (specify whether volunteers or professionals)

Encouragement of involvement in advocacy and fund-raising efforts, including letter writing (list of government officials and sample letter or outline)

PWC "ads": those looking for services, roommates, etc.

Community resources

Humorous articles and cartoons

SUGGESTIONS

A newsletter should not be dominated by the voice of any one individual. That is, the editor should not be writing all the articles, reviewing literature, etc. Ideally, staff should include an editor or coeditors, a reviewer (often a medical reviewer), and someone with a literary background who can proofread articles and make suggestions and corrections (grammar, style, punctuation).

A balance should be maintained among informational articles, editorials and letters to the editor, humor, resources for PWCs, etc. Format is important. A newsletter should be laid out carefully and be easy to read.

The source of each article or information "blurb" should be clearly identified. Obtain permission to use material from other sources. Articles or cartoons found in other CFIDS newsletters, books, and pamphlets may be excellent for your readers and most authors are eager to have you use their material with prior permission. Illustrations add a lot; again, obtain permission if they come from another source.

Newsletters may be brief; most PWCs prefer shorter, more frequent ones. It is an unnecessary duplication of effort to cover topics already covered in national newsletters; a synopsis and suggestion for further reading should suffice.

A Symptom Checklist for CFS

◆

The symptom checklist cannot be used to diagnose Chronic Fatigue Syndrome unless other disorders can be ruled out by physical examination and appropriate laboratory tests.

Rate the severity of your symptoms from 0–10.

____ 1. Fatigue (95%—usually made worse by physical exercise)

____ 2. Cognitive function problems (80%)

    ____ a. attention deficit disorder

    ____ b. calculation difficulties

    ____ c. memory disturbance

    ____ d. spatial disorientation

    ____ e. frequently saying the wrong word

____ 3. Psychological problems (80%)

    ____ a. depression

    ____ b. anxiety—which may include panic attacks

    ____ c. personality changes—usually a worsening of a previous mild tendency

    ____ d. emotional lability (mood swings)

    ____ e. psychosis (1%)

____ 4. Other nervous system problems (75%)

    ____ a. sleep disturbance

    ____ b. headaches

    ____ c. changes in visual acuity

    ____ d. seizures

    ____ e. numb or tingling feeling

    ____ f. disequilibrium

    ____ g. lightheadedness—feeling "spaced out"

    ____ h. frequent unusual nightmares

    ____ i. difficulty moving your tongue to speak

    ____ j. ringing in ears

    ____ k. paralysis

    ____ l. severe muscular weakness

    ____ m. blackouts

    ____ n. intolerance of bright lights

    ____ o. intolerance of alcohol

    ____ p. alteration of taste, smell, hearing

    ____ q. non-restorative sleep

    ____ r. decreased libido

    ____ s. twitching muscles ("benign fasciculations")

___ 5. Recurrent flu-like illnesses (75%)—often with chronic sore throat

___ 6. Painful lymph nodes—especially on sides of neck and under the arms (60%)

___ 7. Severe nasal and other allergies—often worsening of previously mild problems (40%)

___ 8. Weight change—usually gain (70%)

___ 9. Muscle and joint aches with tender "trigger points" or fibromyalgia (65%)

___ 10. Abdominal pain, diarrhea, nausea, intestinal gas—"irritable bowel syndrome" (50%)

___ 11. Low grade fevers or feeling hot often (70%)

___ 12. Night sweats (40%)

___ 13. Heart palpitations (40%)

___ 14. Severe premenstrual syndrome—PMS (70% women)

___ 15. Rash of herpes simplex or shingles (20%)

___ 16. Uncomfortable or recurrent urination—pain in prostate (20%)

___ 17. Other symptoms seen in less than 10% of patients

    ___ a. rashes

    ___ b. hair loss

    ___ c. impotence

    ___ d. chest pain

    ___ e. dry eyes and mouth

    ___ f. cough

    ___ g. TMJ syndrome

    ___ h. mitral valve prolapse

    ___ i. frequent canker sores

    ___ j. cold hands and feet

    ___ k. serious rhythm disturbances of the heart

    ___ l. carpal tunnel syndrome

    ___ m. pyriform muscle syndrome causing sciatica

    ___ n. thyroid inflammation

    ___ o. various cancers (a rare occurrence)

    ___ p. periodontal (gum) disease

    ___ q. endometriosis

    ___ r. easily getting out of breath ("dyspnea on exertion")

    ___ s. symptoms worsened by extremes of temperature

    ___ t. multiple sensitivities to medicine, food and other substances

From the Chronic Fatigue Syndrome Institute, J. A. Goldstein, MD, Director, 500 S. Anaheim Hills Road #128, Anaheim Hills, CA 92807. Some of the above statistics were compiled with the assistance of data provided by Daniel Peterson, M.D., and Paul R. Cheney, M.D., Ph.D.

Bibliography

$\blacklozenge$

BOOKS

Achterberg, J. (1985). *Imagery in healing: Shamanism and modern medicine.* Boston: New Science Library.

Balfour, H. H., and Heussner, R. C. (1984). *Herpes diseases and your health.* Minneapolis: University of Minnesota.

Barry, D. (1988). *Dave Barry's greatest hits.* New York: Crown.

Bell, D. (1991). *The disease of a thousand names.* Lyndonville, NY: Pollard.

Benson, H. (1976). *The relaxation response.* New York: Avon.

Berger, S. M. (1988). *What your doctor didn't learn in medical school . . . and what you can do about it.* New York: Morrow.

Borysenko, J. (1987). *Minding the body, mending the mind.* Reading, MA: Addison-Wesley.

Borysenko, J. (1990). *Guilt is the teacher, love is the lesson.* New York: Warner.

Brooks, B., and Smith, N. (1988). *CFIDS: An owner's manual.* Silver Springs, MD: BBNS.

Conant, S. (1990). *Living with chronic fatigue.* Texas: Taylor.

Cousins, N. (1979). *Anatomy of an illness as perceived by the patient.* New York: Norton.

Cousins, N. (1983). *The healing heart.* New York: Norton.

Cousins, N. (1989). *Head first: The biology of hope.* New York: E.P. Dutton.

Crook, W. G. (1986). *The yeast connection: A medical breakthrough.* New York: Random House.

Elliott, G. R., and Eisdorfer, C. (eds.). (1982). *Stress and human health: Analysis and implications of research.* New York: Springer.

Epstein, M. A., and Achong, B. G. (eds.). (1979). *The Epstein-Barr virus.* New York: Springer-Verlag.

Feiden, K. (1990). *Hope and help for chronic fatigue syndrome.* New York: Prentice Hall.

Ferguson, M. (1980). *The Aquarian conspiracy: Personal and social transformation in the 1980s.* Los Angeles: J.P. Tarcher.

Feuerstein, M., Labbe, E., and Kuczmierczyk, A. (1986). *Health psychology: A psychobiological perspective.* New York: Plenum.

Fisher, G. C. (1987). *Waiting to live: The debilitating effects of chronic Epstein-Barr virus.* Montclair, NJ: Montco, revised and released as *Chronic fatigue syndrome: A victim's guide to understanding, treating, and coping with this debilitating illness.* New York: Warner.

Franklin, M. and Sullivan, J. (1989). *M.E.: What is it? have you got it? how to get better.* London: Century.

Gentry, W. D. (ed.). (1984). *Handbook of behavioral medicine.* New York: Guilford Press.

Gillespie, L. (1986). *You don't have to live with cystitis!* New York: Rawson Associates.

Goldberger, L., and Breznitz, S. (eds.). (1982). *Handbook of stress: Theoretical and clinical aspects.* New York: Free Press.

Goldstein, J. A. (1990). *Chronic fatigue syndrome: The struggle for health.* Beverly Hills, CA: The Chronic Fatigue Syndrome Institute.

Herzlich, C. (1973). *Health and illness: A social psychological analysis.* New York: Academic Press.

Inlander, C. B., Levin, L. S., and Weiner, E. (1988). *Medicine on trial: The appalling story of ineptitude, neglect, and arrogance.* New York: Prentice Hall.

Jeffreys, T. (1982). *The mile-high staircase.* Auckland, New Zealand: Hodder and Stoughton.

Koch-Hattem, A. (1987). Families and chronic illness. In Rosenthal, D. (ed.). *Family Stress.* Rockville, MD: Aspen.

LeMaistre, J. (1985). *Beyond rage: The emotional impact of chronic physical illness.* Oak Park, IL: Alpine Guild.

Levinson, H. L. (1986). *Phobia free.* New York: M. Evans.

Lewis, K. S. (1985). *Successful living with chronic illness.* Wayne, NJ: Avery.

Locke, S., and Colligan, D. (1986). *The healer within: The new medicine of mind and body.* New York: New American Library.

Mizel, S. B., and Jaret, P. (1986). *The human immune system: The new frontier in medicine.* New York: Simon and Schuster.

Monette, P. (1988). *Borrowed time: An AIDS memoir.* New York: Harcourt Brace Jovanovich.

Morozov, P. V. (ed.). (1983). *Research on the viral hypothesis of mental disorders.* Basel, Switzerland: Karger.

Nash, O. (1969). *Bed riddance: A posy for the indisposed.* Boston: Little, Brown.

Pearsall, P. (1987). *Superimmunity: Master your emotions and improve your health.* New York: Fawcett.

Pelletier, K. R. (1977). *Mind as healer, mind as slayer.* New York: Dell.

Pincus, J. H. and Tucker, G. (1974). *Behavioral neurology.* New York: Oxford University.

Pitzele, S. K. (1985). *We are not alone: Learning to live with chronic illness.* New York: Workman.

Podell, R. N. (1987). *Doctor, Why am I so tired?* New York: Pharos.

Randolph, T. G. (1980). *An alternative approach to allergies.* New York: Lippincott and Crowell.

Register, C. (1989). *Living with chronic illness.* New York: Bantam.

Robin, E. D. (1984). *Matters of life and death: Risks versus benefits of medical care.* New York: W. H. Freeman.

Roessler, R., and Decker, N. (Eds.) (1986). *Emotional disorders in physically ill patients.* New York: Human Science.

Rooney, A. A. (1981). Mr. Rooney Goes to Work (orig. broadcast July 5, 1977). In *A few minutes with Andy Rooney.* New York: Warner.

Rooney, A. A. (1982). *Pieces of my mind.* New York: Avon.

Rossi, E. L. (1986). *The psychobiology of mind-body healing: New concepts of therapeutic hypnosis.* New York: Norton.

Schlossberg, D. (ed.). (1983). *Infectious mononucleosis: Praeger monographs in infectious diseases (Vol. 1).* New York: Praeger.

Seligman, M. E. P. (1975). *Helplessness: On depression, development and death.* San Francisco: W. H. Freeman.

Selye, H. (1974). *Stress without distress.* New York: Signet.

Selye, H. (1976). *The stress of life* (rev. ed.). New York: McGraw-Hill.

Shealy, C. N. (1979). *90 days to self health.* New York: Bantam.

Shilts, R. (1987). *And the band played on: Politics, people and the AIDS epidemic.* New York: St. Martin's.

Siegel, B. S. (1986). *Love, medicine and miracles: Lessons learned about self-healing from a surgeon's experience with exceptional patients.* New York: Harper & Row.

Simonton, O. C., Matthews-Simonton, S., and Creighton, J. L. (1984). *Getting well again.* New York: Bantam.

Simonton, S. M. (1984). *The healing family: The Simonton approach for families facing illness.* New York: Bantam.

Solomon, N. (1989). *Sick and tired of being sick and tired.* New York: Wynwood.

Sontag, S. (1977). *Illness as metaphor.* New York: Farrar, Straus and Giroux.

Sontag, S. (1988). *AIDS and its metaphors*. New York: Farrar, Straus and Giroux.

Spink, W. (1978). *Infectious diseases: Prevention and treatment in the 19th and 20th centuries*. Minneapolis: University of Minnesota.

Stearns, A. K. (1984). *Living through personal crisis*. Chicago: Thomas More Press.

Stoff, J. A., and Pellegrino, C. R. (1988). *Chronic fatigue syndrome: The hidden epidemic*. New York: Random House.

Strong, M. (1988). *Mainstay: For the well spouse of the chronically ill*. Boston: Little, Brown.

Trowbridge, J. P., and Walker, M. (1986). *The yeast syndrome*. New York: Bantam.

Viorst, J. (1986). *Necessary losses*. New York: Simon and Schuster.

Watson, M. A., and Sinclair, H. (1986). *Balancing act: For people with dizziness and balancing disorders*. Portland: Good Samaritan Hospital and Medical Center.

Weil, A. (1988). *Health and healing* (rev. ed.). Boston: Houghton Mifflin.

Weil, A. (1990). *Natural health, natural medicine*. Boston: Houghton Mifflin.

Weiner, M. A. (1986). *Maximum immunity*. Boston: Houghton Mifflin.

Wood, T. M. (1989). *Life in the slow lane*. Madison, TN: Woodshed.

PERIODICALS

Adler, T. (1990, July). Neurotoxics called major health threat. *The APA Monitor*, 18.

Adler, T. (1991, February). Optimists' coping skills may help beat illnesses. *The APA Monitor*, 12.

Allen, A. D. (1986, May 3). Epstein-Barr: A causative cofactor [Letter]. *Science News*, 275.

Allen, A. D., and Tilkian, S. M. (1986). Depression correlated with cellular immunity in systemic immunodeficient Epstein-Barr virus syndrome (SIDES). *Journal of Clinical Psychiatry*, 47(3), 133–135.

Altman, L. K. (1990, December 4). Chronic fatigue syndrome finally gets some respect. *The New York Times*.

Amsterdam, J. D., Henle, W., Winokur, A., Wolkowitz, D.M., Pickar, D., and Paul, S. M. (1986). Serum antibodies to Epstein-Barr virus in patients with major depressive disorder. *American Journal of Psychiatry*, 143, 1593–1596.

ANZME Society, Inc. (1991, August). *Meeting-Place 36* [Journal]. Auckland, New Zealand.

Behan, P. O., Behan, W. M. H., and Bell, E. J. (1985). The postviral fatigue syndrome—an analysis of the findings in 50 cases. *Journal of Infection, 10,* 211–212.

Bender, C. E. (1962). Recurrent mononucleosis. *Journal of the American Medical Association, 182* (9), 954–956.

Bennett, W. I. (ed.) (1988, July). Chronic fatigue syndrome. *Harvard Medical School Health Letter,* 1–3.

Berris, B. (1986). Chronic viral diseases. *Canadian Medical Association Journal, 135,* 1260–1268.

Boffey, P. (1987, July 28). Fatigue 'virus' has experts more baffled and skeptical than ever. *New York Times.*

Boly, W. (1987, July-August) Raggedy Ann town. *Hippocrates,* 31–40.

Bothe, K., Aguzzi, A., Lassmann, H., Rethwilm, A., and Horak, I. (1991, August 2). Progressive encephalopathy and myopathy in transgenic mice expressing human foamy virus genes. *Science,* as annotated and excerpted in *CACTUS September 1991 Research Update,* 16–18.

Brigham, C. R. (1988, January). Medical consultant updates: Chronic fatigue syndrome. *LTD Advisor,* Miele and Associates, 12–14.

Brody, J. E. (1985, June 12). An elusive herpes virus makes double misery for its victims. *The New York Times.*

Brody, J. E. (1988, February 16). Personal health: Coping with chronic illness can be grueling in a society that is often blind to the problems. *The New York Times.*

Brody, J. E. (1988, July 28). Personal health: Chronic fatigue syndrome: How to recognize it and what to do about it. *The New York Times.*

Buchwald, D., Cheney, P. R., Peterson, D. L., Henry, B., Wormsley, S. B., Geiger, A., Ablashi, D. V., Salahuddin, S. Z., Saxinger, C., Biddle, R., Kikinis, R., Jolesz, F. A., Folks, T., Balachandran, N., Peter, J. B., Gallo, R. C., and Komaroff, A. L. (1992, January 15). A chronic illness characterized by fatigue, neurologic and immunologic disorders, and active human herpesvirus type 6 infection. *Annals of internal medicine, 116*(2), 103–113

Buchwald, D., Sullivan, J. L., and Komaroff, A. L. (1987). Frequency of 'chronic active Epstein-Barr virus infection' in a general medical practice. *Journal of the American Medical Association, 257,* 2303–2307.

Burden, D. (1989, July/August). Caring for the caregiver. *Psychology Today,* 22.

Caliguiri, M., Murray, C., Buchwald, D., Levine, H., Cheney, P., Peterson, D., Komaroff, A. L., and Ritz, J. (1987). Phenotypic and functional deficiency of natural killer cells in patients with chronic fatigue syndrome. *Journal of Immunology. 139,* 3306–3313.

The CFIDS Association, Inc. *The CFIDS Chronicle.* 1988: February, March, April, June, July, August, September, October, November/December;

1989: January/February, Spring, Summer/Fall; 1990: Spring/Summer, September; 1991: March, Spring, August, Fall.

CFIDS Society International (formerly Chronic Fatigue Syndrome Society and National CEBV Syndrome Society): *The Reporter* (newsletter). 1986: Summer, Fall; 1987: May, July, September; 1988: February, May, July, September, October, November/December; 1989: January; 1990: May; 1991: March.

Chronic fatigue: all in the mind? (1990, October). *Consumer Reports*, 671–675.

Chronic Fatigue Immune Dysfunction Syndrome Foundation (1990, Summer). *CFIDS Treatment News*, 1(1).

Chronic Fatigue Syndrome Association of Arizona (formerly Phoenix Area CEBV Association). *CEBV Jigsaw* (newsletter): 1987: October/ November, December; 1988: February, March, April. *CFS Bulletin* (newsletter): 1988: May, July, August, September, October/November; 1988–89: December/January; 1989: February.

'Chronic mononucleosis' puzzles clinicians. (1987, October 15). *Patient Care*, 19.

Coulter, P. (1988). Chronic fatigue syndrome: An old virus with a new diagnosis. *Journal of Community Health Nursing*, 5(2), 87–95.

Cowley, G. with Hager, M. (1991, September 30). A clue to chronic fatigue. *Newsweek*, 66.

Cowley, G., with Hager, M. and Joseph, N. (1990, November 12). Chronic fatigue syndrome: A modern medical mystery. *Newsweek*, 62–70.

Cowley, G., with Springen, K., Leonard, E. A., Robins, K., and Gordon, J. (1990, March 26). The promise of Prozac. *Newsweek*, 38–41.

David, A. S., Wessely, S., and Pelosi, A. J. (1988, July 9). Myalgic encephalomyelitis, or what? [Letter]. *The Lancet*, 100.

David, A. S., Wessely, S., and Pelosi, A. J. (1988). Postviral fatigue syndrome: Time for a new approach. *British Medical Journal*, 296, 696–699.

De Lisi, L. E., Nurnberger, L. R., Goldin, S., Simmons-Alling, S., and Gershon, E. S. (1986). Epstein-Barr virus and depression [Letter]. *Archives of General Psychiatry*, 43, 815–816.

DeLisi, L. E., Smith, S. B., Hamovit, J. R., Maxwell, M. E., Goldin, L. R., Dingman, C. W., and Gerson, E. S. (1986). Herpes simplex virus, cytomegalovirus and Epstein-Barr virus antibody titres in sera from schizophrenic patients. *Psychological Medicine*, 16, 757–763.

Dengler, R., Thomssen, H., Volkman, M., and Emmerich, B. (1987). Chronic Epstein-Barr virus infection and human immunodeficiency virus infection [Letter]. *Annals of Internal Medicine*, 106, 775.

DuBois, R. E. (1986). Gamma globulin therapy for chronic mononucleosis syndrome. *AIDS Research, 2*(Suppl.1), 191–195.

DuBois, R. E., Seeley, J. K. Brus, I., Sakamoto, K., Ballow, M., Harada, S., Bechtold, T., Pearson, G., and Purtillo, D. T. (1984). Chronic mononucleosis syndrome. *Southern Medical Journal, 77,* 1376–1382.

Edwards, D. D. (1987). Viruses in search of 'compatible' diseases. *Science News, 132,* 246.

Englund, J. A. (1988). The many faces of Epstein-Barr virus. *Postgraduate Medicine, 83*(2), 167–173, 176–180.

Findlay, S. (1988, October 31). New hope for tired people. *U.S. News and World Report,* 71, 73.

Fotheringham, C. (1987, November 18). Tests reveal new clue in fatigue illness. *North Lake Tahoe Bonanza.*

Gantz, N. M. and Holmes, G. P. (1989). Treatment of patients with chronic fatigue syndrome. *Drugs, 38* (6), 856–862.

Gin, W., Christiansen, F. T., and Peter, J. B. (1989). Immune function and the chronic fatigue syndrome. *Medical Journal of Australia, 151,* 117–118.

Goldenberg, D. L. (1990). Fibromyalgia and its relation to chronic fatigue syndrome, viral illness and immune abnormalities. From the Rheumatology, Arthritis-Fibrositis Center, Tufts University School of Medicine, published in *The Mass. CFIDS Update,* Summer, 1990, 27–29.

Goldenberg, D. L., Simms, R. W., Geiger, A. and Komaroff, A. L. (1990). High frequency of fibromyalgia in patients with chronic fatigue seen in a primary care practice. *Arthritis and Rheumatism, 33*(3), 381–387.

Goldstein, J. A. (1986). Treatment of Epstein-Barr virus with H₂ blockers [Letter]. *Journal of Clinical Psychiatry, 47,* 572.

Goldstein, J. A. (1991, January). Chronic fatigue syndrome. *The Female Patient,* 16(1), 39–50.

Greenberg, D. B. (1986). Depression, anxiety, and Epstein-Barr virus infection [Letter]. *Annals of Internal Medicine, 104,* 449.

Grierson, H., Holmes, G. P., and Straus, S. E. (1987, November 15). Coping with chronic fatigue syndrome. *Patient Care,* 79–82.

Hamblin, T. J., Hussain, J., Akbar, A. N., Tang, Y. C., Smith, J. L., and Jones, D. B. (1983). Immunological reasons for chronic ill health after infectious mononucleosis. *British Medical Journal, 287,* 85–88.

Henle, W., and Henle, G. (1981, January). Serodiagnosis of infectious mononucleosis. *Resident and Staff Physician,* 37–43.

Henle, W., Henle, G., and Lennette, E. T. (1979). The Epstein-Barr virus. *Scientific American, 241*(1), 48–59.

Hickie, I., Lloyd, A., Wakefield, D., and Parker, G. (1990). The psychiatric status of patients with the chronic fatigue syndrome. *British Journal of Psychiatry, 156,* 534–540.

Holmes, G. P., Kaplan, J. E., Gantz, N. M., Komaroff, A. L., Schonberger, L. B., Straus, S. E., Jones, J. F., DuBois, R. E., Cunningham-Rundles, C., Pahwa, S., Tosato, G., Zegans, L. S., Purtillo, D. T., Brown, N., Schooley, R. T. and Brus, I. (1988). Chronic fatigue syndrome: A working case definition. *Annals of Internal Medicine, 108,* 387–389.

Holmes, G. P., Kaplan, J. E., Stewart, J. A., Hunt, B., Pinsky, P. F., and Schonberger, L. B. (1987). A cluster of patients with a chronic mononucleosis-like syndrome: Is Epstein-Barr the cause? *Journal of the American Medical Association, 257,* 2297–2302.

Jamal, G. A., and Hansen, S. (1985). Electrophysiological studies in the post-viral fatigue syndrome. *Journal of Neurology, Neurosurgery and Psychiatry, 48,* 691–694.

Jaret, P. (1986). Our immune system: The wars within. *National Geographic, 169,* 702–735.

Johnson, H. (1987, July 16). Journey into fear: The growing nightmare of Epstein-Barr virus [Part 1]. *Rolling Stone,* 56–63, 139–141.

Johnson, H. (1987, August 13). Journey into fear: The growing nightmare of Epstein-Barr virus [Part 2]. *Rolling Stone,* 42–46, 55–57.

Joncas, J. H., Ghibo, F., Blagdon, M., Montplaisir, S., Stefanescu, I., and Menezes, J. (1984, February 1). A familial syndrome of susceptibility to chronic active Epstein-Barr virus infection. *Canadian Medical Association Journal, 130,* 280–285.

Jones, J. F. (1986, October). Epstein-Barr virus: Probable cause of a broad range of infections. *Consultant,* 77–81.

Jones, J. F., Ray, C. G., Minnich, L. L., Hicks, M. J., Kibler, R., and Lucas, D. O. (1985). Evidence for active Epstein-Barr virus infection in patients with persistent, unexplained illnesses: Elevated anti-early antigen antibodies. *Annals of Internal Medicine, 102*(1), 1–7.

Jones, J. F., Shurin, S., Abramowsky, C., Tubbs, R. R., Sciotto, C. G., Wahl, R., Sands, J., Gottman, D., Katz, B. Z., and Sklar, J. (1988). T-cell lymphomas containing Epstein-Barr viral DNA in patients with chronic Epstein-Barr virus infections. *New England Journal of Medicine, 318,* 733–741.

Kaslow, A. (1987, March). Chronic Epstein-Barr virus syndrome. *Let's Live,* 11–12, 14.

Kelly, J. (1988, August). Immunomodulators hailed as Rx. *Medical World News,* 25. (Reprinted in CFS *Bulletin,* CFS Association of Greater Phoenix, December 1988–January 1989).

Klimas, N. G., Salvato, F. R., Morgan, M. and Fletcher, M. A. (1990). Immunologic abnormalities in chronic fatigue syndrome. *Journal of Clinical Microbiology, 28*(6), 1403–1410.

Kohl, R. L., and Lewis, M. R. (1987, December). Mechanisms underlying the antimotion sickness effects of psychostimulants. *Aviation, Space, and Environmental Medicine*, 1215–1218.

Kolata, G. (1990, October). Using body's controls to develop new class of immune boosters. *The New York Times*.

Komaroff, A. L. (1987, May 30). The 'chronic mononucleosis' syndromes. *Hospital Practice*, 71–75.

Komaroff, A. L. (1988). Chronic fatigue syndromes: relationship to chronic viral infections. *Journal of Virological Methods, 21*, 3–10.

Kroenke, K. (1991). Chronic fatigue syndrome: Is it real? *Postgraduate Medicine, 89*(2), 44, 46, 49, 50, 53, 55.

Kroenke, K., Wood, D. R., Mangelsdorff, A. D., Meier, N. J., and Powell, J. B. (1988). Chronic fatigue in primary care: Prevalence, patient characteristics, and outcome. *Journal of the American Medical Association, 270*, 929–934.

Kruesi, M. J. P., Dale, J., and Straus, S. (1989, February). Psychiatric diagnoses in patients who have chronic fatigue syndrome. *Journal of Clinical Psychiatry, 50*(2), 53–56.

Landay, A. L., Jessop, C., Lennette, E. T., and Levy, J. A. (1991, September 21). Chronic fatigue syndrome: clinical condition associated with immune activation. *The Lancet, 338* (8769), 707–712.

Lever, A. M. L., Lewis, D. M., Bannister, B. A., Fry, M., and Berry, N. (1988, July 19). Interferon production in postviral fatigue syndrome [Letter]. *The Lancet*, 101.

Lloyd, A., Hickie, I., Wakefield, D., Boughton, C., and Dwyer, J. (1990). A double-blind, placebo-controlled trial of intravenous immunoglobin therapy in patients with chronic fatigue syndrome. *The American Journal of Medicine, 89*, 561–568.

Lloyd, A. R., Hickie, I., Boughton, C. R., Spencer, O., and Wakefield, D. (1990, November 5). Prevalence of chronic fatigue syndrome in an Australian population. *The Medical Journal of Australia, 153*, 522–528.

Lloyd, A. R., Wakefield, D., Boughton, C., and Dwyer, J. (1988, June 4). What is myalgic encephalomyelitis? [Letter]. *The Lancet*, 1286–1287.

Manu, P., Matthews, D. A., and Lane, T. J. (1988). The mental health of patients with a chief complaint of chronic fatigue. *Archives of Internal Medicine, 148*, 2313–2320.

Marx, J. L. (1985). The immune system 'belongs in the body.' *Science, 227*, 1190–1192.

The Mass. CFIDS Association. *The Update* (newsletter): 1990: Summer, Winter; 1991: Summer.

Masterson, M. (1989, January 29–February 3). The poison within (special series). *The Arizona Republic*.

Murdoch, J. C. (1984). Myalgic encephalomyelitis and the general practitioner. *New Zealand Family Physician, 11*, 127–128.

National Chronic Fatigue Syndrome Association. *Heart of America News* (Newsletter). 1988: September; 1988–89: December/January; Fall/Winter; 1990: Spring/Summer, Fall/Winter.

National Institute of Allergy and Infectious Diseases. (Report: 1990, December). Summary of research on chronic fatigue syndrome (CFS).

National Institute of Allergy and Infectious Diseases. (1988, June). Chronic fatigue syndrome. *Backgrounder*.

National Jewish Hospital for Immunology and Respiratory Medicine. (1984). Epstein-Barr virus. *Med Facts*.

National Jewish Hospital and Research Center; National Asthma Center. (1984). Baffling illness traced to virus. *New Directions, 14*(3).

Nightingale Research Foundation. *The Nightingale* (newsletter). 1989: Fall; 1990: Spring. Ottawa, Canada.

Olson, G. B., Kanaan, M. N., Gersuk, G. M., Kelley, L. M., and Jones, J. F. (1986). Correlation between allergy and persistent Epstein-Barr virus-infected patients. *Journal of Allergy and Clinical Immunology, 78*, 308–314.

Olson, G. B., Kanaan, M. N., Kelley, L. M., and Jones, J. F. (1986). Specific allergen-induced Epstein-Barr nuclear antigen-positive B cells from patients with chronic-active Epstein-Barr virus infections. *Journal of Allergy and Clinical Immunology, 78*, 315–320.

Orbaek, P., and Lindgren, M. (1988). Prospective clinical and psychometric investigation of patients with chronic toxic encephalopathy induced by solvents. *Scandinavian Journal of Work Environment and Health, 14*, 37–44.

Osterholm, K. (1988, January/February). The 10 most hunted viruses. *American Health*, 67–78.

Ostrom, N. (1990). CFIDS: A selected chronology of events. *That New Magazine, Inc.*

Pagano, J. S., Sixbey, J. W., and Lin, J. C. (1982). Acyclovir and Epstein-Barr infection. *Journal of Antimicrobial Chemotherapy, 12*(Suppl. B), 113–121.

Peterson, P. K., et al. (1990). A controlled trial of intravenous immunoglobin G in chronic fatigue syndrome. *The American Journal of Medicine, 89*, 554–560.

Ramsay, A. M. (1976, September). Benign myalgic encephalomyelitis or epidemic neuromyasthenia. *Update*, 539–541.

Ramsay, A. M. (1981, October 7). A baffling syndrome. *Nursing Mirror*, 40–41.

Ramsay, A. M. (1988, July 9). Myalgic encephalomyelitis or what? [Letter]. *The Lancet*, 100.

Salahuddin, S. Z., Ablashi, D. V., Markham, P. D., Josephs, S. F., Sturaenegger, S., Kaplan, M., Halligan, G., Biberfeld, P., Wond-Staal, F., Kramarsky, B., and Gallo, R. C. (1986). Isolation of a new virus, HBLV, in patients with lymphoproliferative disorders. *Science, 234,* 596–601.

Seligman, J., with Abramson, P., Shapiro, D., Gosnell, M., and Hager, M. (1987, Spring). Epstein-Barr: A puzzling virus. *Newsweek, 7.*

South Sound CFIDS Support Group. (1991, April). *South Sound Newsbrief.* Orting, WA.

Spracklen, F. H. N. (1988). The chronic fatigue syndrome (myalgic encephalomyelitis)—myth or mystery? *South African Medical Journal, 74,* 448–452.

Staver, S. (1989, May 26). Meeting sheds light on chronic fatigue. *American Medical News,* 9–10

Steeper, T. A., Horwitz, C. A., Henle, W., and Henle, G. (1987). Selected aspects of acute and chronic infectious mononucleosis and mononucleosis-like illnesses for the practicing allergist. *Annals of Allergy, 59,* 243–250.

Stewart, D. E. (1986). Environmental illness and patients with multiple unexplained symptoms [Letter]. *Archives of Internal Medicine, 146,* 1447.

Straus, S. E. (1987). EB or not EB—that is the question [Editorial]. *Journal of the American Medical Association, 257,* 2335–2336.

Straus, S. E. (1988). The chronic mononucleosis syndrome. *Journal of Infectious Diseases, 157,* 405–412.

Straus, S. E., Dale, J. K., Tobi, M., et al. (1988). Acyclovir treatment of the chronic fatigue syndrome: Lack of efficacy in a placebo-controlled trial. *New England Journal of Medicine, 319,* 1692–1697.

Straus, S. E., Tosato, G., Armstrong, C., Lawley, T., Preble, O. T., Henle, W., Davey, R., Pearson, G., Epstein, J., Brus, I., and Blaese, R. M. (1985). Persisting illness and fatigue in adults with evidence of Epstein-Barr virus infection. *Annals of Internal Medicine, 102*(1), 7–16.

Sumaya, C. V. (1977). Endogenous reactivation of Epstein-Barr virus infections. *Journal of Infectious Diseases, 135*(3), 374–379.

Swartz, M. N. (1988). The chronic fatigue syndrome—One entity or many? [Letter]. *New England Journal of Medicine, 319,* 1726–1728.

Tobi, M., David, Z., Feldman-Weiss, V., (1982, January 9). Prolonged atypical illness associated with serological evidence of persistent Epstein-Barr virus infection. *Lancet,* 61–64.

Tobi, M., and Straus, S. E. (1985). Chronic Epstein-Barr virus disease: A workshop held by the National Institute of Allergy and Infectious Diseases. *Annals of Internal Medicine, 103,* 951–953.

Tosato, G., Straus, J., Henle, W., Pike, S. E., and Blaese, R. M. (1985). Characteristic T-cell dysfunction in patients with chronic active

Epstein-Barr virus infection (chronic infectious mononucleosis). *Journal of Immunology, 134*, 3082–2088.

Trubo, R. (1986, May 12). Viruses: The lurking menace. *Medical World News, 56–58*, 63–71.

Turkington, C. (1985, November). Viruses tied to mental symptoms. *Monitor*, American Psychological Association, *16*(11).

Wakefield, D., Lloyd, A., Dwyer, J., Salahuddin, S. Z., Ablashi, D. V. (1988, May). Human herpesvirus 6 and myalgic encephalomyelitis [Letter]. *The Lancet*, 1059.

Weikel, W. J. (1989, May). A multimodal approach in dealing with chronic Epstein-Barr viral syndrome. *Journal of Counseling and Development, 6*, 522–524.

Wilber, K., and Wilber, T. (1988, September/October). Do we make ourselves sick? *New Age Journal*. (Reprinted in *CFS Bulletin*, CFS Association of Greater Phoenix, 1988–89, December/January).

Winslow, R. (1991, September 16). Virus may have role in causing chronic fatigue. *The Wall Street Journal*, B1, B2.

Zarski, J. J., West, J. D., DePompei, R., and Hall, D. E. (1988). Chronic illness: Stressors, the adjustment process, and family-focused interventions. *Journal of Mental Health Counseling, 10*, 145–158.

Zoler, M. L. (1988, December 12). Chronic fatigue: Taking the syndrome seriously. *Medical World News, 33–41*.

OTHER

Archard, L. (1990, February). Molecular virology of muscle disease: Persistent virus infection of muscle in patients with post-viral fatigue [lecture]. Los Angeles: Chronic Fatigue Syndrome and Fibromyalgia: Pathogenesis and Treatment.

Bastien, S. (1991, May 19). Neuropsychological deficits in CFS [lecture]. Bel Air, CA: CFS: Current Theory and Treatment.

Behan, P. (1990, February). Recent findings in patients with post-viral fatigue syndrome [lecture]. Los Angeles: CFS and FM: Pathogenesis and Treatment.

Bell, D. (1987, November 6). Outbreak of chronic fatigue syndrome in New York State [lecture transcript]. Wilsonville, OR: National CEBV Convention.

Bell, D. (1988, October). Lecture presented at the Rhode Island CFIDS Symposium [audiotape].

Bell, D. (1990, February). Chronic fatigue syndrome in children: The role of symptom severity rating [lecture]: Los Angeles: CFS and FM: Pathogenesis and Treatment.

Buchwald, D. and Mease, P. (1990, February). Chronic fatigue syndrome and fibromyalgia: Current research findings and treatment approaches [lecture]. Los Angeles: CFS and FM: Pathogenesis and Treatment.

Caro, X. (1990, February). Is there an immunologic component to the fibrositis syndrome? [lecture]. Los Angeles: CFS and FM: Pathogenesis and Treatment.

The Centers for Disease Control (1990, January). The chronic fatigue syndrome: An information pamphlet.

The CFIDS Association, Inc. In *The CFIDS Chronicle* (1991, Spring). Unravelling the mystery: The CFIDS Association research conference [transcript].

Cheney, P. R. Diagnostic criteria for C.E.B.V. syndrome [information sheet]. Incline Village, NV.

Cheney, P. R. (1987, January 13). An outbreak of chronic fatigue illness characterized by fatigue, neurologic, and immunologic disorders: Epstein-Barr virus, cause or effect? [videotape]. Reno, NV: Washoe Medical Center.

Cheney, P. R. (1987, January 14). Chronic Epstein-Barr virus syndrome [audiotaped lecture]. Incline Village, NV.

Cheney, P. R. (1987, November 5). Definition of chronic fatigue syndrome: Causes, health concerns. Is this a real entity? [lecture transcript]. Wilsonville, OR: National CEBV Association Convention.

Cheney, P. R. (1987, November 7). Closing comments: Final remarks concerning chronic fatigue syndrome [lecture transcript]. Wilsonville, OR: National CEBV Association Convention.

Cheney, P. R. (1988, October). Lecture presented at the Rhode Island CFIDS Symposium [audiotape].

Cheney, P. R. (1990, February). Chronic fatigue syndrome: An immunological perspective [lecture]. Los Angeles: CFS and FM: Pathogenesis and Treatment.

Cheney, P. R. (1991, May 18). CFS: A current perspective [lecture]. Bel Air, CA: CFS: Current Theory and Treatment.

DeFreitas, E., Hiliard, B., Cheney, P., Bell, D., Kiggundu, E., Sankey, D., Wroblewska, Z. and Koprowski, H. (1990, September). Evidence of retrovirus in patients with chronic fatigue immune dysfunction syndrome [presentation at 11th International Congress of Neuropathology]. Kyoto, Japan.

De Freitas, E. (1991, November 13). Chronic fatigue syndrome: Diagnosing the doubt [teleconference]. CTV World Television.

Demitrack, M. (1991, November 13). Chronic fatigue syndrome: Diagnosing the doubt [teleconference]. CTV World Television.

Fudenberg, H. H. (1990, February). Immunotherapy of chronic fatigability immune dysregulation syndrome [lecture]. Los Angeles: CFS and FM: Pathogenesis and Treatment.

Goldenberg, D. (1990, February). A controlled study of tender points in patients with chronic fatigue syndrome [lecture]. Los Angeles: CFS and FM: Pathogenesis and Treatment.

Goldstein, J. A. (1987, November 6). The psychoneuroimmuno-pharmacology of the chronic fatigue syndrome [lecture transcript]. Wilsonville, OR: National CEBV Association Convention.

Goldstein, J. A. (1988, October). A unified hypothesis of CFIDS: Pathophysiology, diagnosis, and treatment. [lecture audiotape]. Rhode Island CFIDS Symposium.

Goldstein, J. A. (1990, February). Presumed pathogenesis and treatment of the chronic fatigue syndrome/fibromyalgia complex [lecture]. Los Angeles: CFS and FM: Pathogenesis and Treatment.

Goldstein, J. A. (1991, May 18). Limbic encephalopathy in a dysregulated neuroimmune network [lecture]. Los Angeles: CFS: Current Theory and Treatment.

Goldstein, J. A. (1991, May 19). Medical management of the CFS patient in family practice [lecture]. Bel Air, CA: CFS: Current Theory and Treatment.

Grufferman, S. (1987, November 5). CEBV controversy: What we need to do to gain credibility in the research world and with the general public [lecture transcript]. Wilsonville, OR: National CEBV Association Convention.

Gunn, W. (1991, November 13). Chronic Fatigue syndrome: Diagnosing the doubt [teleconference]. CTV World Television.

Hallowitz, R. (1988, October). Lecture presented at the Rhode Island CFIDS Symposium [audiotape].

Handleman, M. J. (1990, February). Neurological substrates of behavior: Brain mapping and the chronic fatigue patient [lecture]. Los Angeles: CFS and FM: Pathogenesis and Treatment.

Herberman, R. B. (1990, February). Abnormalities in immune system in patients with chronic fatigue syndrome [lecture]. Los Angeles: CFS and FM: Pathogenesis and Treatment.

Hermann, W. (1990, February). Inhibition of T-cell mitogen response in chronic fatigue syndrome [lecture]. Los Angeles: CFS and FM: Pathogenesis and Treatment.

Hyde, B. (1990, February). The definition and history of ME/CFS [lecture]. Los Angeles: CFS and FM: Pathogenesis and Treatment.

Hyde, B. (1991, May 18). A report on the NIH consensus conference redefining CFS [lecture]. Bel Air, CA: CFS: Current Theory and Treatment.

Iger, L. M. (1990, February). The MMPI as an aid in confirming a chronic fatigue syndrome diagnosis [lecture]. Los Angeles: CFS and FM: Pathogenesis and Treatment.

Iger, L. M. (1991, May 19). Cognitive restructuring with the CFS patient [lecture]. Bel Air, CA: CFS: Current Theory and Treatment.

Imperati, S. (1987, November 6). Social security disability: A lawyer's view [lecture transcript]. Wilsonville, OR: National CEBV Association Convention.

Jacobson, E. (1991, May 18). Drug therapy in CFS: A psychobiologic approach [lecture]. Bel Air, CA: CFS: Current Theory and Treatment.

Johnson, A. (1987, November 6). Environmental factors and their effect on chronic fatigue syndrome [lecture transcript]. Wilsonville, OR: National CEBV Association Convention.

Jones, J. F. (1987, February 4). Sinequan used as treatment for symptoms of CEBV [memorandum]. Denver: National Jewish Center for Immunology and Respiratory Medicine.

Jones, J. F. (1988, October). Lecture presented at the Rhode Island CFIDS Symposium [audiotape].

Jones, J. F., and Cheney, P. (1986, June). Chronic Epstein-Barr virus [videotaped lecture]. Lake Tahoe, NV.

Jones, J. F., and Hutter, M. J. (1983). Instructional guide to chronic Epstein-Barr infection [transcript of videotaped lecture]. Tucson, AZ: Biomedical Communications.

Khalsa, G. S. S. (1987, November 6). Naturopathic medicine: Applications in chronic viral illness [lecture transcript]. Wilsonville, OR: National CEBV Association Convention.

Komaroff, A. (1988, October). Lecture presented at the Rhode Island CFIDS Symposium [audiotape].

Komaroff, A. (1991, November 13). Chronic fatigue syndrome: Diagnosing the doubt [teleconference]. CTV World Television.

Levinson, H. (1987, November 7). Cerebellar-vestibular dysfunction and phobias [lecture transcript]. Wilsonville, OR: National CEBV Association Convention.

Levinson, H. (1987, November 6). Introduction to balance disorders [lecture transcript]. Wilsonville, OR: National CEBV Association Convention.

Lloyd, A. R. (1990, February). The pathophysiology of "fatigue" in patients with chronic fatigue syndrome [lecture]. Los Angeles: CFS and FM: Pathogenesis and Treatment.

Lloyd, A. (1991, November 13). Chronic fatigue syndrome: Diagnosing the doubt [teleconference]. CTV World Television.

Lottenberg, S. (1990, February). Positron emission tomography in chronic fatigue syndrome [lecture]. Los Angeles: CFS and FM: Pathogenesis and Treatment.

Loveless, M. O. (1987, November 7). Chronic fatigue syndrome: A post-viral immunologically mediated disease? [lecture transcript]. Wilsonville, OR: National CEBV Association Convention.

Loveless, M. O. (1991, May 18). Chronic immunologic activation and CFS [lecture]. Bel Air, CA: CFS: Current Theory and Treatment.

Martin, W. J. (1990, February). Detection of viral sequences using the polymerase chain reaction [lecture]. Los Angeles: CFS and FM: Pathogenesis and Treatment.

Mena, I. (1990, February). Study of cerebral perfusion by NeuroSPECT in patients with chronic fatigue syndrome [lecture]. Los Angeles: CFS and FM: Pathogenesis and Treatment.

Mena, I. (1991, May 18). Study of cerebral perfusion by NeuroSPECT in patients with CFS [lecture]. Bel Air, CA: CFS: Current Theory and Treatment.

Minann, Inc. Statistical data on diagnosed patients [unpublished study]. Glenview, IL.

Moldofsky, H. (1990, February). The significance of sleep-wave physiology and immune functions to chronic fatigue syndrome and fibromyalgia [lecture]. Los Angeles: CFS and FM: Pathogenesis and Treatment.

National Cancer Institute, Office of Cancer Communications. (1986, October). NCI isolates new human herpes-like virus. Cancer Facts.

National CEBV Syndrome Association, Inc. Guidelines for interpreting EBV antibody titers [report]. Prepared with the help of James F. Jones, M.D., Denver: National Jewish Center for Immunology and Respiratory Medicine.

National CFS Association. Chronic fatigue syndrome [brochure]. Kansas City, MO.

National Institute of Allergy and Infectious Disease. (1991, November 12). NIAID funds three CFS cooperative research centers. Update.

Nightingale Research Foundation (Spring, 1990). The Cambridge symposium on Myalgic Encephalomyelitis (M.E.): Summary of proceedings.

Nord Disease Database (1986, May 1). Information on CMV [report].

Peterson, D. (1991, May). Phoenix, AZ: Lecture given at monthly meeting of The CFS Association of Arizona.

Peterson, D. (1991, May 18). Progress report of Ampligen 2-5A study [lecture]. Bel Air, CA: CFS: Current Theory and Treatment.

Peterson, D. (1991, November 13). Chronic fatigue syndrome: Diagnosing the doubt [teleconference]. CTV World Television.

Reed, J. C. (1988, March). Treating CEBV [lecture]. Phoenix, AZ: monthly meeting of the CFS Association of Arizona.

Ross, J. (1987, November 7). How CEBV patients can win social security disability benefits [lecture transcript]. Wilsonville, OR: National CEBV Association Convention.

Rubin, P. (1988, September 6). Phoenix, AZ: Lecture given at monthly meeting of the CFS Association of Arizona.

Russell, I. J. (1990, February). Fibrositis syndrome: Diagnosis, pathogenesis and management [lecture]. Los Angeles: CFS and FM: Pathogenesis and Treatment.

Sandman, C. (1990, February). Is there a CFS dementia? [lecture]. Los Angeles: CFS and FM: Pathogenesis and Treatment.

Sandman, C. (1991, May 18). How CFS affects memory [lecture]. Bel Air, CA: CFS: Current Theory and Treatment.

Schluederberg, A. (1988, May). Information on research conducted by the National Institute of Allergy and Infectious Diseases (NIAID) on chronic Epstein-Barr (CEBV) infection and chronic fatigue syndrome (CFS). NIAID: Bacteriology and Virology Branch, Microbiology and Infectious Diseases Program.

Sleight, R. B. (1988, October). Lecture presented at the Rhode Island CFIDS Symposium [audiotape].

U.S. Department of Health and Human Services (1991, December 2). HHS News.

Wakefield, D. (1990, February). Immunological abnormalities and immune therapy in chronic fatigue syndrome [lecture]. Los Angeles: CFS and FM: Pathogenesis and Treatment.

Index

ORDER FORM

10% DISCOUNT on orders of $20 or more —
20% DISCOUNT on orders of $50 or more —
30% DISCOUNT on orders of $250 or more —
On cost of books for fully prepaid orders

NAME

ADDRESS

CITY/STATE   ZIP

COUNTRY (outside USA)   POSTAL CODE

TITLE	QTY	PRICE	TOTAL
The New A-to-Z of Women's Health		@ $ 16.95	
The A-to-Z of Women's Sexuality		@ $ 14.95	
The Enabler		@ $ 6.95	
Getting Pregnant & Staying Pregnant		@ $ 12.95	
Healthy Aging *(soft cover)*		@ $ 11.95	
Healthy Aging *(hard cover)*		@ $ 17.95	
Lupus: My Search for a Diagnosis		@ $ 6.95	
Menopause Without Medicine *2nd Edition*		@ $ 12.95	
Once A Month *4th Edition*		@ $ 9.95	
Running on Empty *(soft cover)*		@ $ 13.95	
Running on Empty *(hard cover)*		@ $ 21.95	

Shipping costs:
First book: $2.00 ($3.00 for Canada)
Each additional book: $.50 ($1.00 for Canada)
For UPS rates and bulk orders call us at (510) 865-5282

TOTAL
Less discount @_____%   (   )
TOTAL COST OF BOOKS
Calif. residents add sales tax
Shipping & handling
TOTAL ENCLOSED
Please pay in U.S. funds only

❏ Check   ❏ Money Order   ❏ Visa   ❏ M/C

Card # _____ Exp date _____

Signature _____

Complete and mail to:
Hunter House Inc., Publishers
2200 Central Ave. Ste. 202, Alameda CA 94501-4451
Phone (510) 865-5282 Fax (510) 865-4295

❏ Check here to receive our book catalog

RMT 03/92